MY PULSE

IS NOT WHAT IT USED TO BE

The Leadership Challenges
In Health Care

Irwin M. Rubin, Ph.D.
President, The Temenos® Foundation

C. Raymond Fernandez, M.D.
Medical Director, Nalle Clinic

The Temenos® Foundation
Honolulu

First Edition

Designed by Momi Cazimero, Graphic House, Inc.

Library of Congress Cataloging in Publication Data

Rubin, Irwin M.
    My Pulse Is Not What It Used to Be: The Leadership Challenges in Health Care.

  1. Management. I. Fernandez, C. Raymond. II. Title

ISBN 0-9629561-0-4

DEDICATION

Na kahuna lapa'au (Hawaiian):
"Expert practitioners who cure illness"

THE PRACTICE of medicine is in an unhealthy and costly state of disease. Suspicion and mistrust have infected the sacred nature of the doctor-patient relationship. As a result, the central issue facing the profession of medicine is "how we [doctors] will respond to the challenges of public accountability for quality: with anxiety, reluctance and defensive action, or with confidence, enthusiasm, and a sense of pride . . . ."[1]

This book is dedicated to the growing body of physicians in management, *na kahuna lapa'au,* whose patients needing quality care are organizations of providers. We hope that by reading its message, they will draw the experience, strength, and hope that they require to move forward with confidence, enthusiasm, and pride. The success of their effort is vitally important, for at some point in our lives, we are all touched by the practice and business of medical care.

---

[1] Dr. Donald Berwick, "Measuring Health Care Quality," *Pediatrics in Review,* 10, no. 1 (July 1988), p. 16.

ACKNOWLEDGMENTS

THIS BOOK is intended to be a message of hope—massaging the heart and feeding the soul—as well as stimulating the mind and engaging the intellect of a badly beleaguered profession. Given that vision, it comes as little surprise that this final section has been harder for me to draft than any other. Letting go of a baby I've come to hold near and dear to my heart is (as Dr. Fernandez writes), emotionally painful.

I feel a parental sense of both incompleteness ("I know it could be better"), and pride ("I can't believe how it has grown"), as well as a sense of gratitude that mere words cannot convey. Bruce Fritch, Keith Korenchuk, Gail Fernandez, and Drs. Kevin Sullivan and John Benedum have generously added essential perspectives. In addition to writing his own insightful commentary, Dr. Henry Berman has functioned as an invisible co-author throughout. Without his emotional and substantive support, I might have taken the easier, softer way out upon occasion and settled for less from myself.

When my ego resistance to Henry's help remained firm, my trusted editors, first David Nelson and then Tracey Bennett, would rise to the challenge. Tracey, in particular, had the remarkable ability to hang in with me long enough so that I could finally let go and say what I meant.

When all else failed, standing beside me and getting through my ego's defensiveness, as she has done with love and care since the day we met, is my partner and best friend, Nancy Holmes.

Readers will be privileged to get to know and appreciate for themselves Dr. Ray Fernandez. There are qualities of the man that only face-to-face contact can provide. While this book is about Charles Ray Fernandez as a personality, it is a tribute to him that his motivation and commitment have, throughout, been in support of a principle. Treating people in the most humane way possible is a fact of life for Ray Fernandez. Equally unshakable is his faith in the fundamental goodness of our human nature.

Without Dr. Ray Fernandez and his profession and the principles they represent, this book, and message of hope that it carries, would remain the mere vision of an idea. At some point in our lives we are all touched by the practice and business of medical care, and we all owe it a measure of grateful acknowledgement.

Irwin Rubin
Honolulu
March 1991

TABLE OF CONTENTS

CASE PRESENTATION:
MEDICAL RECORD

Patient's Name: The Nalle Clinic

Attending Physician: Raymond Fernandez, M.D., CEO

Chief Complaint:

Increasing overhead, trouble making decisions, poor morale

Presenting Illness:

*T*his 70-year-old multi-specialty clinic with nearly 80 physicians is located in a medium-sized southern city. From its inception, it has enjoyed progressive growth and an excellent regional reputation as a quality medical provider, notably of specialty care. More recently, it has expanded its primary care base. For years it had an extremely low rate of physician attrition. It was quite financially successful through the 1970's.

The Clinic's home city of Charlotte, North Carolina, has grown steadily. The physician community doubled between 1985 and 1990. Local hospitals expanded and began competing with one another and with physician groups. In 1984 HMO's entered the community, and in only five years, expanded from zero to fifteen percent penetration. As these competitors began to market physicians' services, then competition and advertising, unheard of ten years previously, became standard.

Several specialty groups left the Clinic, including the entire nephrology and cardiology sections and major components of the orthopedic and gastroenterology sections. Hiring high-earning subspecialists became quite difficult. Small niche groups were enjoying more financial success in the community than this large multi-specialty group. Members began to question the compensation formula that had served the Clinic for 60 years. This formula, based on production, consisted of an equal-percentage contribution by all physicians. Some began to advocate cost accounting with its appealing variable contribution to overhead. Over a five-year period, two separate committees wrestled with a new compensation formula, but neither committee could get a new formula accepted.

Between 1985 and 1990 the Clinic changed its expensive computer system twice. Physicians grumbled more and more about reports from the data processing department, and eventually they began to disbelieve most reports. The percentage that physicians recognized of their billings continued to decline, as did the collection percentage. Although all physicians demanded "better management," their disdain for bureaucracy and administration intensified. Physicians did not volunteer to serve on the Board of Directors. Rather, like Monday morning quarterbacks, many knew exactly what plays should have been called. Few seemed willing to leave their seats on the 50-yard line and join the battle on the astroturf.

Past Medical History:

In spite of escalating problems, the Clinic recorded numerous successes. It reobtained three-year accreditation from the AAAHC. The Clinic's HMO quickly grew to 35,000 members, the most successful in the region. Over the most recent five-year period, the Clinic added three new satellites; began a seven-day, extended-hour, acute-care facility; dedicated a CT scanner; initiated a women's specialty center with five physicians; and hired a marketing director. The number of patient visits continued to rise. In 1980 the Clinic introduced the role of medical director, and four years later, it established the role of CEO. On the level of national successes, a member of the Clinic has served as the President of the American Group Practice Association. Another of the Clinic's members went on to serve as President of the American Academy of Medical Directors.

In spite of many signs of good health, and in spite of improvements in the physicians' benefit package, the Clinic's debt load skyrocketed.

Review of Systems:

Managerial The Clinic recognized that one person could not handle the administrative load. Previously, only one lay administrator had been responsible for the whole Clinic. The Clinic replaced this arrangement with a physician-CEO and an administrative team of newly hired professionals.

Data Processing Twice the Clinic completely changed the computer system and the personnel who operated it between 1985 and 1990.

Morale Members of the Clinic acknowledged, and attrition and turnover figures confirmed, that morale of both physicians and employees was declining.

Financial The Clinic's line of credit with its bank increased dramatically. For the first time, the Clinic established a capital reserve fund, but could not adequately fund it. Increased debt load made borrowing funds difficult, even for operations.

Recruitment Recruitment became difficult, especially of the high earners. For the first time, the Clinic had to employ recruitment firms.

Decision Making Members of the Clinic frequently appealed the decisions made by the Board and committees. Lengthy delays in making and implementing decisions became common. The Clinic never did implement certain decisions. Over a five-year period, two separate committees studied cost accounting, but the Clinic's members would not accept any of their proposals.

Physical (Objective) Examination:

Physicians' salaries and benefits decreased to approximately 43 percent of collected dollars.

Over a three-year period, the value of a share of stock in the Nalle Clinic diminished significantly.

Personnel turnover was averaging more than 20 percent per year.

Physicians who left were increasingly difficult to replace, and some positions lay vacant for long periods, resulting in significant problems with patient access.

HMO growth had stagnated at 35,000, and the Clinic stopped all marketing efforts because of inability to provide primary care to any more prepaid patients. In 1989 the fee-for-service equivalency on prepaid activities fell to less than 75 percent.

Diagnostic Work-Up and Initial Treatment Plan:

Editor's note: The diagnostic work-up and initial treatment plan that Dr. Fernandez implemented are the subject of the case report which follows.

OVERVIEW OF
THE CASE REPORT

by Irwin Rubin, Ph.D.

W hen a physician becomes the CEO of a health-care organization, the entire organization becomes that physician's patient, and the physician takes on a role we will refer to as *physician-CEO*. Other physicians provide essential leadership and managerial expertise formally in their roles as medical directors, chiefs of service, and department heads, and informally in their day-to-day practices. While these individuals may or may not have the well-being of the entire organization in mind when they act, a physician-CEO must always have the well-being of the organization in mind. The case that follows concerns such a physician, such an organization, and the changes and growth that both are experiencing.

The five-year period of the chart entries we are about to examine is but a slice in time in the 70-year history of a proud organization. We emphasize that this is *not* the story of a terminally-ill organization trying to save itself. Rather, this is the story of a normal patient-organization experiencing normal growing pains in a stressful environment. It is a story that thousands of health-care organizations are living at this very moment. In whatever form it is destined to grow, the institution will continue to be a living, breathing force searching for excellence in patient care.

The search for excellence is the foundation of the entire profession of medicine. Continuous improvement in quality care rests on publishing the results of intensive scrutiny of clinical cases. The classic method of case reports allows the sharing of experiences of successes and failures. This sharing helps the profession progress by allowing new generations to share the hard-earned knowledge of their predecessors without suffering through the pain of having to learn the same lessons in the same hard way. An array of hard new lessons present themselves daily as learning opportunities. Continuous improvement through experiential learning is critical, perhaps even more so when the patient is an entire organization of providers.

In the chart we are about to review, one such physician, Dr. Raymond Fernandez, and one such organization, the Nalle Clinic, courageously open their medical records for public scrutiny. (We will not include any information of a purely private or proprietary nature.) By allowing us a glimpse into the human nature of their encounters—as provider and patient—Dr. Fernandez and the Nalle Clinic are contributing to the changes and growth that an entire industry and its captains are experiencing. The opportunity to learn from their experience, without critical judgment, is a rare gift.

The case presentation has four parts. Following the outline of a typical patient work-up, Part One contains some of Dr. Fernandez's reflections, thoughts and feelings about the historical events leading up to his accepting the role of physician-CEO of the Nalle Clinic. This material is an edited version of a book chapter published in September 1988.[2]

Dr. Fernandez's and the Nalle Clinic's experiences reflect the massive developmental changes confronting the entire health-care industry. As each major chart entry will, Part One closes with a commentary. The intent of these commentaries is to stimulate you, the readers who share a common concern for improving the quality of patient care. The core of this first commentary is an article I published in 1987: "Organizations Have to Grow Up"[3] describes the stages of growth through which all health-care organizations, the Nalle Clinic being a single clinical example, must progress as they mature.

Having noted the patient's chief complaint and presenting symptoms, scanned its medical record, and reviewed elements of its history, we move to an examination of Dr. Fernandez's diagnostic work-up and initial treatment plan. Part Two offers us a glimpse of the patient's and provider's private medical records. Three memos, or chart entries, that Dr. Fernandez sent to his patient let us study leadership in action in organizational cultural change.

The anonymous questionnaire and open-group discussion that Dr. Fernandez refers to in the first memo reflect an X-ray diagnosis of his patient's initial state of health. These chart entries in Part Two will provide two things: first, a feel for the process of surveying a patient-organization's human climate and, second, a glimpse of the issues and insights crucial to deciding on a treatment plan.

Each of these chart entries freezes a moment in time: an encounter between a patient-organization and its physician-CEO. These chart entries represent the first series of official interactions between patient and doctor. As such, they offer insights into the psychological contracting between the physician-CEO and his patient-organization. This relationship mirrors the dynamics of early encounters between patients in pain and the providers they depend on for relief. Memos such as these give us insights into *what* physician–CEO's do and *how* they go about their practice.

Readers searching for formulas and therapies may find these chart entries and subsequent commentary incomplete. Just as each patient is unique, so is a patient-organization. We will highlight general patterns and processes, not quick-fix solutions. Leadership in organizational cultural change requires the flexible and humane application of generic healing therapies to each organization.

Part Three contains the edited transcripts of a tape Dr. Fernandez dictated and

---

[2] Charles Raymond Fernandez, "Personal Managerial Evolution in a Multispecialty Clinic," *Roads to Medical Management*, ed. Wesley Curry, (Tampa: AAMD, 1988), pp. 74–77.

[3] "Organizations Have to Grow Up," *Physician Executive*, 13, No. 2, (March–April 1987), pp. 2–6.

sent to Dr. Rubin on December 5, 1988. These personal chart entries give us a progress report of Dr. Fernandez's feelings some four years into his CEO relationship with his patient-organization. The patient was experiencing predictable growing pains. The feelings Dr. Fernandez reports will enhance the logic and rationality of his first-person, historical introduction to Part One.

In addition to Dr. Rubin's commentaries, Part Three includes commentaries from five guest lecturers. Dr. Henry Berman, President and CEO of Group Health Northwest, is a seasoned veteran of the challenges of having an entire organization as his patient. Dr. Kevin Sullivan, current Vice President of Medical Affairs of Port Huron Hospital, whose commentary follows Dr. Berman's, is a potential candidate for a position as physician-CEO. While Dr. Sullivan is responsible for a significant piece of his organization, he does not, unlike Dr. Berman, occupy the seat where the buck stops. The commentaries of these two respected physicians, each at different stages of their own careers as leaders of organizational cultural change, add unique perspectives to the material Dr. Fernandez provides.

The final progress-report commentaries in Part Three speak to the shifting nature of the relationships between and among the central participants in the process of growing up. Keith Korenchuk, partner in the law firm of Parker, Poe, Adams & Bernstein, has served as the Nalle Clinic's attorney since 1982. His observations on the changing nature of legal issues—for example, stock ownership and restrictive covenants—balance the psychological contracting that has been our focus. Dr. John Benedum is President of the Nalle Clinic Board and a long-standing friend and colleague of Dr. Fernandez's. Through his eyes we see the patient's view of the cultural change which occurred. Bruce Fritch is a consultant with extensive experience with organizations; his recent clients include the Nalle Clinic. His third-party insights concerning the shifting nature of the balance of power between physicians and patients have enormous implications for the entire health-care industry. Based on discussions with Mr. Fritch, Dr. Rubin added a commentary to Part Three: "Turbulent Passages of Change and the Dynamics of Power."

The chart entry in Part Four, the final section of this case, consists of newspaper articles and portions of taped conversations that occurred between January 31 and March 5, 1990, between Dr. Fernandez and his wife, Gail Fernandez. During this period the Nalle Clinic completed its current stage of development, and Dr. Fernandez's role as physician-CEO came to a close. As we shall be privileged to see in Part Four, Dr. Fernandez's feelings resonate more deeply and intensely as a natural, though often painful, part of the leadership of organizational cultural change.

While the facts and circumstances surrounding Dr. Fernandez's stepping down as physician-CEO in March 1990 have significance for him, his family, and the Nalle Clinic, we will not discuss them here. As a result, some will find the case incomplete. However, our objective is not to judge success—either of Dr. Fernandez as physician-CEO or of the Nalle Clinic as an organization. Our objective is to identify, and learn from, some of the generic dynamics of leadership and organizational cultural change, particularly in the beginning and penultimate phases.

The final two commentaries in Part Four bring us full circle with our patient workup. In "What's It All About, Alfie?" dated August 1990, Dr. Fernandez offers his prognosis. He addresses the questions "What does all this change and its effect on me [as attending physician] and the organization [as my patient] really mean?" and "What are the lessons here?" In "Human Parallels to Organizational Development" Dr. Rubin offers his prognosis of what this case suggests are the challenges faced by the health-care industry as it struggles in search of excellence in patient care.

We hope these commentaries and the entire case will encourage you to discuss your own experiences as physician and non-physician managers striving to bring the highest ideals of patient care to the practice of medicine.

Finally a word about the title we have chosen for the book. We call attention to *The Leadership Challenges* because its capital letters spell out TLC. While there is value to be drawn from D.R.G.'s (Diagnostically Related Groups), losing sight of the healing power of TLC could prove to be our most costly mistake. The most powerful ingredient of quality care cannot be commandeered or bought. Neither is it the sole responsibility of doctors and nurses. By caring for one another, every person in a provider organization has the power to contribute to the creation of a healing culture.

We are all equal partners in meeting the leadership challenges in health care.

Part One:

History

HISTORICAL EVENTS CHART ENTRY

by Dr. Raymond Fernandez
September 1988

I know of no school for physician-CEO's. To my knowledge, no educational curriculum alone can prepare one for this role. Thus, I offer my description of my experiences as the first Medical Director and Chief Executive Officer of the Nalle Clinic in the hope that it will help bridge some gaps for others in health care who have accepted, or are considering accepting, leadership roles.

The Nalle Clinic, a private, multi-specialty group in Charlotte, North Carolina (population 500,000), has existed since 1921. I joined the Clinic in 1975 as an internist and infectious-disease specialist. In less than 15 years, it has grown more than in its previous 55 years, doubling from 40 to nearly 80 physicians. This expansion and the many environmental changes facing medicine in general have greatly increased the complexity of the organization, changing a big small clinic into a small big clinic. Currently the Clinic is making the transition from condominium orientation (physicians sharing facilities but running their own practices) to a team approach to the delivery of medical care.

In 1978 the only administrative leadership role for a physician at the Nalle Clinic was President of the Board of Directors. The physician whom the Board elected President received neither compensation for the position nor time to perform the duties of the office. At that time, a task force studying whether the Clinic should have a medical director rejected the position as a "waste of a physician's time."

However, critical duties such as recruiting physicians, planning for the future, and disciplining physicians began to demand an inordinate amount of the President's time. Finding people to serve on the Board was also becoming difficult because of the commitment those duties required. In 1981 the Board recognized that important decisions were taking too long because the President's decision-making capacity was not adequate, and therefore decided to elect a physician to a management position as medical director. The medical director was to devote 50 percent of his time to administrative matters at a salary of 50 percent of the average Clinic physician's income. The idea was to financially motivate the medical director to improve the physicians' incomes.

The relationship of this new medical director to the non-physician administrative team was unclear. The Board did not spell out the position's power and authority, except to point out that the medical director would attend Board meetings in an advisory capacity but would not vote. The job description included such duties as planning, developing agendas for Board and committee meetings, communicating, and recruiting. Clearly, the medical director would need strong interpersonal, communication, problem-solving, and public-relations abilities.

When the Board elected me the Clinic's first Medical Director, one of my highest priorities was to obtain some type of training to give me the necessary background for my new position. Fortunately, one of the physicians in our group was active in the American Academy of Medical Directors (now the American College of Physician Executives) and pointed me toward its management courses. Programs from the American Group Practice Association, the Medical Group Management Association, and the American Management Association also helped me to understand my new role. The Clinic provided an allowance to promote my education. However, as I believe everyone expected, most of my learning experience was on-the-job training and consisted of learning quickly from mistakes I made along the way.[4]

By 1983 I realized that 50 percent of my time was not adequate to perform all the duties of medical director and that I was also shortchanging my patients. The Board readily agreed to my suggestion that I devote 85 percent of my time to the medical director's duties. This change required that I give up all of my internal medicine practice, although I was able to keep my infectious disease consultant's role relatively unchanged. Because I went off the call schedule,[5] members of my department who now had to cover for me faced increasing demands on their time. But at this point we all realized that my primary role had changed from being a clinician to being an administrator.

At a series of planning retreats in late 1984 and early 1985, the Board of Directors established a corporate structure for governing the Clinic. The Board staked out its authority to make decisions—even the tough, unpalatable ones. It designated for the first time the role of the chief executive officer, who would be in charge not only of the physician matters, now the duty of the medical director, but also of administrative matters. The CEO was to be the boss of the administrators as well as of the physicians. The Board invited me to accept that role.

---

[4] *Editor's note:* Dr. Fernandez's motivation and willingness to learn on the job can be seen, in part, from the changing nature of the titles prominent in his own library. Prior to 1985, Starr's *The Social Transformation of American Medicine*, Meisenheimer's *Quality Assurance*, and Roberts' *Rules of Order* were prime examples. A current review of his well-used library would uncover Peters, et al.'s *Thriving On Chaos* and *A Passion for Excellence*, Goldsmith's *Can Hospitals Survive?*, and Walton's *The Deming Management Method*.

[5] My call schedule hasn't changed since I took action to leave the Internal Medicine call schedule in 1983. I am on Infectious Disease call rotation—every 3–4 days; 1–3 consultations (each taking approximately 1 hour) in the hospital after regular work hours. Every fourth weekend I make hospital rounds and answer consults on Sat. and Sun. for 3 partners, which takes 4–8 hours per day on those days.

COMMENTARY:
ORGANIZATIONS HAVE TO GROW UP

by Irwin Rubin, Ph.D.

A health-care organization is a living, breathing, human organism. There are hands-on providers and support personnel. Everyone, including management, is a semi-permanent member. This human healing organism—a hand-holding company—is the patients' contact when they visit this culture. Economically and humanely, the more temporary the patients' visit, the better.

As a consequence of their humanness, health-care organizations—like every social system—will reflect the entire range of human experience: they will go through good times and tough times. Right now the organized practice of medicine is dis-eased. Suspicion and mistrust characterize the provider-patient relationship. As a prerequisite to healing this relationship, to growing up, organizational cultures providing care will have to first heal themselves.[6]

Every institution is born from the seed of an idea. Like parents, its founding entrepreneurs put up with many sleepless nights and colicky outbursts. And, like a child, an organization proceeds through predictable developmental phases. As someone's entrepreneurial baby struggles for an identity of its own, for the chance to grow beyond its biological and emotional roots, we can expect growing pains.[7] If the CEO is inhumanely replaced, the organization may suffer a trauma as frightening as a flood of crushing chest pains. And not all organizations or industries will survive. Stronger corporate cells often take over, sometimes in a hostile way, organizations unable to learn from their experience and grow up. As the steel and automobile industries can attest, proud institutions do become extinct.

Organizations progress through a series of stages as they grow. How they handle themselves in each stage will determine how rapidly they progress to new stages, and whether they succeed to a new stage at all. Those organizations that adjust to growth most effectively become the standard setters that other organizations follow. We conceive, build, maintain, inhabit, and, when it is ill, heal, the human organism we call a health-care organization.

There are three categories of issues that any organization, like the Nalle Clinic,

---

[6] The initiation and management of this healing process will be led by physicians. The phenomenal growth of organizations such as the American College of Physician Executives confirms the fact that many physicians are preparing themselves to face the challenges of leadership in organizational cultural change.

[7] Decision-making dynamics are related to a team's age profile: therefore, individual's mid-life crises can not be kept from the meeting room.

must address: mission, structure, and procedure. It is the responses to these issues and the processes by which the responses are made visible that define an organization's stage of development. The degree of alignment determines effectiveness in any stage of development: does form (structure) fit with function (mission), and are both supported and reinforced by procedures?

Mission: Every organization exists for a purpose. It has a mission, a direction, written or unwritten. As a result, a psychological contract operates between individual members and the organization. This contract defines what individuals can expect to get and what they are expected to give. The contract is balanced when individuals' and the organization's missions overlap.

Many mission statements are more rhetoric than reality. Consequently, the operational mission must often be inferred from behavior. It is important to emphasize that the focus here is on how the organization really operates, not on what appears in a formal statement. The Nalle Clinic's mission, as we shall see in Part Two, reflected a combination of desire and reality.

Structure: At its most basic level, the issue of structure involves questions of power. Who has what powers and upon what basis? As Dr. Fernandez has noted, "Important decisions were taking too long because the President's decision-making" power was no longer adequate. Structural changes were necessary. The formal organizational chart will be relevant, but it will not be the entire picture. An informal structure will develop: organizational bypasses will compensate for plugged arteries.

As was true with the mission, the operational structure most often will be inferred from observable patterns of behavior. Particularly important will be patterns that develop around the management of differences, the organization's response to conflict. Conflict situations represent arenas where individuals play out an organization's legitimized power games. For example, there are status pecking orders in group-practice settings, with "real-doctor" surgeons at the top and general practitioners, family doctors, and "couldn't-hack-it-in-medical-school" psychiatrists lower down. Psychiatrists who care for the worried well and physicians who treat flu symptoms are more valued by their patients than by their organizational colleagues. These pecking orders will be reflected in the organization's power structure.

Procedures: The underlying purpose behind any organizational procedure is to increase the probability that individuals' behaviors will support the mission. The procedures by which an organization recruits, selects, and orients new members can, if aligned with the mission, attract people who already fit into the organization.

Key among these procedures is the organization's system of "consequence management." At issue here are the processes intended to address performance appraisals, rewards and punishments. There is also the issue of individual and organizational development via training, career development, and organizational succession. How does the organization strive to guide the behavior of members? The initial process of reviewing these structures and procedures at the Nalle Clinic began at a series of planning retreats in late 1984 and early 1985.

Before describing the three stages of organizational development, I want to emphasize the generic quality of these issues. Any two people who expect to develop and sustain a relationship must come to some agreement, often implicit, as to their mission in life. Their psychological contract speaks to what each can hope to get and will have to give to realize their common mission. The lack of agreement as to what constitutes "goodness," "quality," or "success"—mission-related issues—is the source of much conflict in intimate relationships.

Each couple—for instance, man and wife—will develop its own power structure. As men's and women's roles diverge from stereotypical roots, couples often find themselves at odds: she wants to explore her own career interests; he wants her to stay at home.

Mundane, day-to-day tasks essential to survival must be allocated and completed. Taking out the trash, scrubbing the bathrooms, and balancing the checkbook, while not as glamorous as performing rare surgical procedures, are pieces of the business of living. Each couple needs to resolve its conflicts ("All right. This Thanksgiving we'll go to your mother's. But we'll spend Christmas with my dad"), to make unpopular decisions, and to complete unappealing chores.

As with individuals and organizations, couples move through various stages of development. The exhilarating "no-one-else-exists-in-the-world-but-us," care-free glow of the honeymoon period passes into the need to grow up, to get down to the business of taking life one day at a time.

Now let's look at the three stages of organizational development.

STAGE 1: THE FRATERNITY MODEL

Many health-care organizations, group practices in particular, are remarkably similar to college fraternities. Individual freedom of expression is the central driving force. Each person is highly committed to selfish special interests (e.g., area of study). The primary reason for being together is not task interdependence.

Individual member commitment is time-bounded (e.g., four years at college). Dues will be paid "as long as I get what I want." This fraternity orientation feeds, and is consistent with, a mind set of low tolerance for delayed gratification. In psychological terms, the fraternity-model organization stimulates and feeds what Maslow called lower-order human needs. The primary focus is on self-satisfaction and personal security. Goodies—such as money, time off, and trips to professional-development meetings in Hawaii and Bermuda—like food on the frat dinner table, are grabbed by those with the longest reach and quickest hands.

Mission Issues: Regardless of what the written version may be, the operational mission of a fraternity-model health-care organization is the satisfaction of individual member's and/or owner's needs. The organization exists to satisfy the immediate needs of its most powerful members. Individuals give up some security and opportunities for synergy. In return, they get relatively high degrees of individual freedom and minimal organizational control. In its most extreme form, the mind set is one of "renting space from the administrative entity" with all the consequent grumbling about overhead.

Structure Issues: A health-care organization at this stage of development is replete with a host of we-they dynamics: physicians mistrust administrators; surgeons look askance at family practitioners; nurses align themselves with their doctors; and founding seniors tolerate "young Turks."

Formal role constraints are minimal. Indeed, the formal organization charts are quite flat, particularly on the medical side. Physician managers are often figureheads, with more administrative than managerial responsibilities. They are more reactive than proactive.

Where stock ownership is a factor, a variety of blackball dynamics show up. The board regularly finds hours of hard work overturned by a single stockholder. Professional, non-physician administrators defend themselves against stockholders who bemoan how "their" hard-earned dollars are being spent. It should come as no surprise that conflict avoidance pervades the organization.

Procedures: A high degree of randomness and/or lack of selectiveness characterizes the new membership process. Often, a new member is the friend of a current member, and trial memberships of varying lengths are typical before someone achieves what amounts to tenure.

Many a fraternity-model health-care organization is surprised at how many behavior problems show up shortly after a new member becomes a stockholder. Such a turn of events should surprise no one; the absence of such examples would be a surprise. Individuals rushing a fraternity are on their good behavior during hazing. Behavior problems are unlikely to surface until after the ritualistic induction into the brotherhood.

Systems of formalized performance appraisal, if they exist at all on the medical side, focus exclusively on broad standards of patient care. Similarly, in a fraternity individuals enjoy wide behavioral boundaries. All manner of acting out is tolerated as long as it does not threaten the basic sanctity of the brotherhood. That is, it is all right to get drunk and rowdy at parties as long as neighbors don't call the police. Constraints on personal behavior in fraternity-like organizations are virtually nonexistent, as is any formalized reward-and-punishment system, short of termination.

Given the fraternity orientation, short-range income concerns consume the organization. Members spend hours designing and reworking salary formulas. Even more energy is spent in maintaining the system by those who benefit, in reaction to those who feel shortchanged. Almost everyone gets a chance to be in each group more than once.

Organizationally supported development is infrequent or nonexistent. Time for professional development might be granted if the production formula takes this time into account. Organizational development for physicians taking on managerial responsibilities receives token financial support and even less emotional support.

STAGE II: THE BASIC BUSINESS ORGANIZATION

If a Stage-I organization is characterized by a childlike orientation, Stage II is akin to a young-adult orientation. The underlying theme is "Let's get serious, let's get down to business." Degrees of task interdependence are accepted. Delayed gratification becomes a tolerated reality.

The organization's long-term investment strategies reflect this expectation. There will be reserves set aside for new facilities to ensure the continuing growth and replacement of the physical plant, although individuals who are holding on to the Stage-I fraternity mentality will resist having to sign their names to long-term mortgage notes for new facilities. There will be new retirement programs allowing individuals to defer income to later stages of their personal life-cycles. Organizational contributions and vesting conditions are often hotly contested issues.

The design and implementation of these longer-term investment strategies require careful planning. Like the Stage-II organizational culture in which they are embedded, they are intended, in psychological terms, to stimulate and feed Maslow's middle-level needs for belonging and self-esteem. But to those who are more comfortable in a fraternity-type organization, golden parachutes can become golden handcuffs. Individuals who feel imprisoned by long-term promises can become embittered, poisoning their own and others' senses of belonging and self-esteem.

Mission Issues: The operational mission of a Stage-II organization is survival, adaptation, and growth in its external market environment, which is hostile and competitive. The organization's formal mission, if it exists, focuses on achieving short-term results, such as improving the fee-for-service vs. HMO-income ratio by x% and decreasing billing times.

The operating psychological contract shifts accordingly. People give up some individuality and accept more organizational control. In return, they get the security offered by an organization and the attendant economies of scale. The mind set is "You work for, and are protected by, the organization." This has a much higher level of psychological commitment than simply "renting space." Consequently, the structure is different.

Structure Issues: While power differences still exist, they are somewhat less imbalanced, the degree varying according to the strength and maturity of the organization. The basic hierarchical model remains the underlying structure in Stage II. Loose, informal boundaries of Stage I are replaced by very careful, formalized role descriptions. The medical side of the organization, while still relatively flat, now has physician managers with varying degrees of positional power and personal training.

Blackball dynamics have given way, often grudgingly, to more democratic actions. In the strongest Stage-II organizations, decision-making protocols ("who is to be involved?" "how?" in "what decisions?"), have become formalized procedures that minimize the day-to-day squabbles of the fraternity model.

Resolving conflicts is essential, so avoidance is no longer the dominant orientation. Minimizing emotional heat remains the primary unspoken objective. Compromising (resulting in both parties being half-satisfied) or forcing (by those with the positional power to do so) become the dominant modes of conflict management.

Procedures: The importance of the organization, its need to outlive any single member, manifests itself in more rationalized systems of recruitment, selection, and orientation. The organization hires professional search firms. Personnel applying for jobs may have to take psychological tests. *What* you know and *what* you've done become more important than *who* you know.

In the most mature Stage-II organizations, formalized performance appraisal systems begin to appear *throughout* the organization. Only a small number of Stage-II health-care organizations step up to the need to define and assess the interpersonal behaviors of their physician members. Indeed, the way in which Stage-II organizations handle this procedural issue will be a major factor in their movement into, and level of growth within, this stage of organizational development.

Income will remain an important concern. Mature Stage-II organizations develop mechanisms to depersonalize and rationalize the process. This means a formula must be agreed upon. It will tie individual salaries to measurable behaviors deemed relevant (at least in theory), to the achievement of the agreed-upon mission. While the result may be a mechanistic, impersonal formula, the process of designing the formal reward system will be emotionally charged and personal. At this point the day-to-day meaning of the mission's words on paper come to life.

How much is it worth to the organization, to that elusive commodity called quality care, to see one more patient/hour versus scheduling slack time so patients can talk? How much is it worth to inconvenience the physicians by having full evening and weekend office coverage versus meeting patients' needs for access? "My short-term income as a practitioner may drop if we hire a new physician now. On the other hand, patients may not need to wait months for an appointment."

In designing their compensation formula, Stage-II organizations are putting their money where their mouth is. Little wonder that enormous numbers of hours go into the design of the compensation system. In the most mature form of the Stage-II organizations, once hashed out, the issue is (with the exception of minor adjustments), put to bed. In contrast, members of the immature Stage-II organizations, like fraternity members, return to this formula and try to squeeze out more for themselves every chance they get.

Whereas fraternity-model organizations spend little on individual and/or organizational development, Stage-II organizations do invest in such programs. Medical management, for example, becomes valued enough to develop and pay for, even though the attitude about it is still defensive. But when the external environment gets tough, a Stage-II organization will typically seek to cut its development budget.

MOVING FROM STAGE I TO STAGE II

It is important that we examine what conditions are necessary for an organization to consciously move from Stage I to Stage II. Strengthening these conditions will enhance an organization's growth as a Stage-II entity.

The Mechanics of the Shift: The organizational mechanisms needed to move from Stage I to Stage II are not the least bit mysterious. A mission statement focusing on clear, concise, quantitative goals is the starting point. Then monitoring systems, planning functions, and formal statements of authority and responsibility can be designed to attain mission goals.

At the procedural level, the key issue revolves around the performance-appraisal system. It makes absolutely no sense to develop an organizational mission if performance appraisal is to be left as an abstraction. People need to know what they are expected to do. These behaviors need to be agreed upon, defined, measured, and fed back.

While help may be gained from outside the organization, the final answer—what equals "good behavior"—must come from within. The unwillingness and inability of a health-care organization to step up to this issue, particularly as it relates to physicians (who may also be owners), keeps many at Stage I or ensures that growth within Stage II is stymied. (The same is true of individuals. As we struggle to grow up, we increasingly take responsibility for our own behavior.)

In the extreme, this is the procedure that decides ultimately whether a single individual is bigger than the organization. There will be instances in which a "bottom-line" decision must be made on a very high-income producer who refuses, or is unable, to behave in harmony with the mission.

Hostage high-jacking dramas are played out with frightening regularity. Because of specialty and extraordinary technical competence, for example, a surgeon may generate millions of dollars in gross revenues, not to mention a hefty personal income. On many occasions this same physician regularly exhibits behaviors that fall, if not outside the letter of the mission, certainly outside its spirit. For example, a physician schedules a golf game and tells a nurse to cancel a patient's appointment. If the nurse, the front-line provider of TLC, questions these priorities, the nurse may be verbally abused by the prima-donna high earner.

A 1990 court ruling in San Antonio, Texas,[8] drove home the financial, not to mention professional, implications of an organization's contributing to hostage dynamics. A patient's malpractice suit involved a host of other physicians as accomplices because it could be proven that they knew her physician—their colleague—was impaired and not delivering quality care. The $5 million settlement ought to send a much-needed message as to the real bottom-line decisions confronting the profession.

The Underlying Attitude Behind the Shift: The major attitude shift in moving from Stage I to Stage II has to do with the perceived value of the organization and management. For a successful transition to Stage II, the managerial function must be believed to *add value* as opposed to being seen as an overhead expense. The seriousness of this belief system will be seen, or not, in the way the organization selects, trains, rewards, and otherwise supports its managers, whose responsibility, in turn, is to ensure that all of the organization's assets—human and otherwise—are effectively and efficiently aligned with the mission.

As a consequence, some individuals will not want, or be able, to stay. Many will have consciously joined a fraternity model and only be happy in that form of organization. As humanely as possible, they need to be helped to find an environment that better fits their needs.

How long should such a transition from Stage I to Stage II take? Absolute numbers are impossible to provide. A minimum of 3–5 years would not be surprising. The resources involved to cover *expected* and *necessary* training to support the development of new behavioral patterns, not needed in Stage I, will be extensive. The amount will be a function of how long the organization has been in Stage I and how strong a Stage-II organization it hopes to become.

STAGE III:
AN ORGANIZATION IN SEARCH OF EXCELLENCE

A Stage-III organization has a mature-adult orientation. The organization and its members have a holistic orientation. Everyone feels empowered by task interdependence. The resulting need for high-level teamwork is not considered a necessary evil.

Consequently, individual members thrive on challenge, trust, change, and innovation. In psychological terms, a Stage-III organization meets all of Maslow's lower-order/middle-order needs and stimulates and feeds higher-order needs for self-

---

[8] James E. Schutte, "An Impaired Doctor Cost His Colleagues $5 Million," *Medical Economics*, (June 4, 1990), pp. 45–50.

actualization. The required shift in mind set is dramatic, as one would expect, given the potential benefits to be realized. It is a quantum leap, *not* a mere extrapolation.

Mission: The mission of a Stage-III organization steps beyond merely reacting to a basically hostile external environment. This organization strives to be a standard setter that Stage-II organizations follow. The organization's formal mission, which will certainly appear on paper, focuses on the achievement of long-term, hard-to-measure, *qualitative* values. One such organization, on the verge of beginning a continuing search for excellence, unashamedly and sincerely has the words *love, joy,* and *nurturance* in its mission statement.

The operating psychological contract for a Stage-III organization is unique and expensive. The organization provides security from arbitrary layoffs, but not from dismissal for continued unacceptable performance. It also provides regular opportunities for challenge, autonomy, and synergy. In return, individual members are expected to give up a piece of their *souls*—to invest their *selves* in the business.

The mind set of Stage-III people is "I am the organization." When numerous individuals feel as if the organization is *their* business, they attend carefully to their investment. It is rational selfish behavior with win-win consequences.

Structure: In such a psychological climate, we note a significant change in the power dynamics. No longer is rigid hierarchy necessary or relevant. Personal power is more important than formal position. The mission, not turf battles, is paramount. Organizations in search of excellence are both "tight and loose." As Peters and Waterman have so carefully documented,[9] they are fluid.

Given the inadvisability of always relying on "the boss" to resolve conflicts, individuals are required to develop a win-win orientation. They confront their differences within the powerful common ground afforded by the organization's mission. Pooling and sharing all income, increasingly common among forward-thinking groups and departments, is a far cry from the me-first grabbing that characterizes a Stage-I mentality.

What keeps people on track? The rigid hierarchical structure of a Stage-II organization tells people that they need supervision. But the operating structure of an organization in search of excellence relegates control to a trust-based *SUPER VISION.*

Procedures: We talk easily of "the system" as if it were a God-given entity rather than a creation of our minds. Stage-III organizations know better. They know that organizations in search of excellence are made of *individuals* who are in search of excellence, and that self-actualizing individuals will create self-actualizing organizations. Organizations in search of excellence put enormous energy into recruitment,

---

[9] Thomas J. Peters and Robert H. Waterman, Jr., *In Search of Excellence*, (New York: Harper & Row, 1982), pp. 318–325.

selection, and orientation. They try to help people to self-select. For example, one very large high-tech organization in search of excellence requires, by its mission, people who see themselves as innovative entrepreneurs. The opening line in its new-hire advertisements announces that "Digital Equipment (DEC) is looking for *individual contributors* in the area of . . . ." Many candidates react with the thought, "Individual contributor? All I want is a job!" DEC breathes a sigh of relief as one unlikely fit self-selects out!

With respect to orientation, Disney World provides other organizations with food for thought. A summer employee who works for only 10 weeks gets five days (10%!) of orientation training. At the end of that period, if the mission requirement of treating all customers as "guests in someone's home" has not been internalized, the candidate is released.

Organizations in search of excellence recognize that everyone has "customers." A boss has subordinates as customers. Numerous formal and informal mechanisms exist to ensure that everyone gets customer feedback. Rather than fear this continual feedback, members seek and thrive on it. These organizations recognize that as individuals grow and develop, the organization will, too. IBM, a clear standard setter in this regard, invested over $1 billion in 1985 to support the development of its 300,000 employees. The 40,000 people who wear the mantle "manager" must, by IBM's requirements, take two weeks of management development each year. When the external environment gets tough, Stage-III organizations typically seek to *increase* their development budgets.

I would like to illustrate how one health-care organization treats its members and its patients "as guests in someone's home."

Because she is the first person visitors meet when they enter the lobby, the official greeter is one of the most important and respected persons at St. Marguerite Hospital, Chiba, Japan. So vital is her role to the success of the business that her position requires a minimum of ten years of experience as a nurse. The woman who greeted me on March 2, 1988, was in her late 50's and had been a nurse for more than 30 years. As I soon learned, this attention to the human component of quality care permeates St. Marguerite.

My official host was 60-year-old Dr. Seiichi Satoh. The previous day, he had participated in a seminar I conducted on health-care management in the U.S. He said that he would be honored if I would visit his hospital. He was eager to learn all he could to help his hospital.

St. Marguerite's mission is simple and straightforward. To paraphrase Dr. Satoh, "Although people do not wish enthusiastically to go to the hospital, if they must go, we intend to have them choose happily to consult St. Marguerite." The hospital's brochure promises total medical service, high tech and human touch, hand in hand in pursuit of St. Marguerite's goal: to provide quality care and quality life in a resort atmosphere on a foundation of human kindness. The words embossed on the plaque outside the front door introduce the promise:

To heal sometimes
To support often
To comfort always

The hospital cares well for its healthy elderly. An elevator-like stretcher lowers the incapacitated into the warm-water bath so culturally critical to the cleansing of their bodies and souls. Along with an Olympic-size pool (the kindest exercise), and fla- menco dance (great for flexibility), St. Marguerite provides English lessons because many patients wish to visit the U.S. before they die. The hospital planned to break ground soon for a hospice.

In the dormitory-style hospital rooms, ample breathing space between the six beds is the norm. For those who can afford them, private rooms are available. The hospi- tal also provides space for family members to sleep, with either futon or Western- style beds.

The secret of St. Marguerite Hospital is no secret at all. It's the same message that has been available to us from the Japanese for years. Our own excellence research has uncovered similar truths, which we all reacted to as being common sense. Still, we have yet to explain why such common sense is so uncommon a reality. The key to excellence begins and ends with how the staff treat one another.

I asked Dr. Satoh how St. Marguerite's management had inculcated human kind- ness into the organization. (A professional staff of 8 full-time and 13 part-time physi- cians and 70 nurses forms the core of the total staff of 160 at St. Marguerite. Five peo- ple hold full-time managerial positions.) Careful selection of staff was the start, he said, but just the start. For the six months prior to the opening of the new, expanded services in October of 1987, which took the hospital from 200 beds to 315, the two most senior managers, including the equivalent of a Western medical director, spent the better part of every day walking around St. Marguerite, talking to the staff about the importance of kindness. We call this ritual MBWA, management by walking around, and it's a ritual they perform with daily regularity and undocumented impact.

To his answer I can only add my own observations. The respect Dr. Satoh showed all the other staff was, in one sense, purely Japanese. Arriving on a floor, we first stopped at the nurse's station. Without my daughter and son-in-law along to inter- pret, I would have followed right on Dr. Satoh's heels, not understanding his request that I wait a moment. Before taking us onto a floor, several of which were still empty, Dr. Satoh needed to announce and explain our presence and to request permission to enter. Dr. Satoh, a most senior physician, requested permission to enter! A warm- ly smiling nurse or nurse's aide scurried along beside us in case we required any assistance. We could examine equipment, even if it was not in use, only after Dr.

Satoh had briefed the attending physician.

I didn't understand any of the conversations between Dr. Satoh and the people with whom he spoke during my tour. Despite the best efforts of my daughter and son-in-law to translate, we missed many of the words. But respect and kindness transcend the boundaries of language and culture. In a way that is consistent with their culture, the people of St. Marguerite Hospital afforded me and one another immeasurable respect and kindness. They have much to teach us about how to turn common sense into common human service.

THE QUANTUM LEAP

If it does make great sense to treat human resources in a Stage-III manner, we must ask, "Why do few organizations venture out of the security of Stage II to embark on a search for excellence?" We hypothesized that the implicit mission of a Stage-II organization is survival, adaptation, and growth within a basically competitive, hostile, external market environment. So the resultant formal mission statement emphasizes short-run quantitative goals. As a result, an organization develops an emphasis on *not losing*.

An organization in search of excellence has made a conscious choice to move to a higher plane than its Stage-II colleagues. Given the need to engage people's souls, a mission that reaches deeply into untapped human potential must be formulated. This means focusing on deeply held values. The collective mind set is upon winning something that really matters to people's souls, a dramatically different attitude from "not losing." Within a mind set of winning, there are no mistakes. There are only valuable learning experiences.

The mentality of *doing whatever needs to be done* is crucial to the search for excellence. An organization will have to design its own new structures and procedures continuously. Successes will fuel the motivation to move to the next plateau of achievement. As customers and members get used to excellence, their standards go up. To meet rising expectations, managers will have to invent new solutions. Yesterday's success will be the training ground for tomorrow's challenge, not necessarily the answer to tomorrow's challenge.

This mentality is infinitely easier to write about than to implement. It flies in the face of much managerial folklore and practice. "If it ain't broke, don't mess with it" is one such attitude, and it may minimize losing. At the same time, it ensures minimal innovation. Managerial practice and education are long on problem solving—hunting down and rooting out causes of mistakes—and frightfully short on success management—identifying and spreading out causes of successes. Organizations in search of excellence know better, which is why they function better.

The toughness that develops while succeeding in Stage II provides the strength to venture into Stage III. But success is not guaranteed. Success during Stage II depends primarily upon the depth and quality of managerial talent available. Managers are responsible for "doing things right." They focus on keeping the organization on course. Management by objectives, MBO, captures the essence of this responsibility.

Entering and succeeding in Stage III requires acts of leadership. Whereas a Stage-II manager focuses on "doing things right," a Stage-III leader focuses on the question, "What is the right thing to do?" Rather than being a play on words, these phrases represent two dramatically different mind sets. The natural tension between them is the hallmark of an organization in search of excellence. It is the constant tension between "Who are we? How are we doing?" and "Who could we be? How could we get there?"

APPLICATION TO THE NALLE CLINIC

Let's turn from a description of the three stages to our study of the Nalle Clinic. The Nalle Clinic, as the patient-organization and Dr. Fernandez, as its physician-CEO providing the needed guidance, met formally when the patient was in its mid-sixties. In chronological terms, the patient-organization was not young. In developmental terms, it mirrored a Stage-I fraternity model. (The Clinic's term was "medical condominium.") The Clinic wanted to change its mind set to that of a Stage-II basic business organization. To accomplish this, members of the Clinic would have to change their commitment from "I rent space from an administrative entity" to "We work for the organization, and it protects us."

In developmental terms, the patient's chief complaint, presenting illness, and past history all suggest a gangling adolescent struggling to grow beyond its childhood. The teenager learns that not only does he live in a house with his family, he must act as a team member with his siblings and parents. In the same way, the physicians needed to change their orientations from, as Dr. Fernandez put it, "physicians sharing facilities, but running their own practices" to "a team approach to medical care." The search for excellence forces us to continuously decide *what* we want to be when we grow up and *how* to get there.

Many balk at the notion of excellence: "It is an ideal! It can never be achieved!" Their dilemma is one of perspective: they see "it"—excellence—as a specific, finite place where we arrive; they don't see it as the quality of the journey we are all on. In that sense we never grow up; instead we are continuously in the process of growing up. The dissatisfaction and emptiness many successful senior executives feel at the peak of their careers reflects the processes used (or abused) in getting to the top. For example, many executives missed their child's second birthday party or their first little-league home run. In short, they traded time with their families for time with their careers. And then they feel lonely at the top. The nature and quality of our process of growing up will determine the success we experience along the way.

Like that of a rebellious adolescent, the patient-organization's initial posture toward management and leadership, toward care from its providers, was a 50-50 split. The appointment of a medical director who was "to devote 50 percent of his time to administrative matters at a salary of 50 percent of the average Clinic physician's income" replaced zero compensation for the "waste of a physician's time."

Human nature seeks to have its cake and eat it, too. Humans expect to be cured without taking responsibility for their own wellness. Placing unclear lines of authority and power in the hands of a person whose medical training has not given him the strong interpersonal communication, problem-solving, and public-relations abilities necessary for success has the earmarks of an impossible mission. The fact that physicians dominate the patient-organization complicates this mission in several ways.

Patients tend to give up too much power to their doctors, treating them like gods. Physicians, on the other hand, have great difficulty relinquishing control under any circumstances, particularly when they are in the patient role. Organizational cultural change will shift the balance of power away from individual physicians. In a similar vein, many of the members of the Nalle Clinic grew up professionally during the golden age of physician power, 1955 to 1985. The sense of entitlement they developed is shifting uneasily as the entire medical profession matures. Doctor-driven organizations will regularly present their physician-CEO's with the challenges of managing non-compliant patients.

Leadership in organizational cultural change requires intuitive and formal skills. Fortunately, educational support was available for Dr. Fernandez. Still, he expected—as he believed others did—that most of his learning would be experiential, "from mistakes [he] made along the way."

By 1983 the 50-50 bargain was more than Dr. Fernandez could tolerate. His integrity was at stake: "I realized that 50 percent of my time was not adequate to perform all the duties of medical director and that I was also shortchanging my patients." A major emotional and cognitive shift was necessary: he had to devote all his time to one patient, an entire organization of care-providers.

In late 1984 the Board invited Dr. Fernandez to quarterback the Nalle Clinic's life-support team during a period of transition. The Board invited him to accept the role of CEO, "the boss of the administrators as well as the physicians." It was a role for which no job description existed; it was a role without a school, other than experience, to learn from.

What Dr. Fernandez did and said—his style of communication—and how he provided life support, technically and humanely, were the tools of his practice as he struggled to care for his patient-organization. As a physician-CEO, he had to learn to act honorably, with persistence.

In Part Two, we examine through three early chart entries, concrete manifestations of this reality.

Diagnostic Work-Up and Initial Treatment Plan

CHART ENTRY

Memo to:	**All Staff**
From:	**CEO**
Date:	**December 13, 1984**
Subject:	**Nalle Clinic Organization Workshop**

*T*wo weekends ago, the Board of Directors met in a retreat and made decisions that will have significant implications for all members of the Nalle Clinic family. The Board is redefining the mission of the Clinic.

A seminar that Dr. Irv Rubin conducted this past weekend helped members of the Clinic analyze, not only our strengths, but also our weaknesses. Not only physicians and administrators but several people representing other employees of the Clinic attended this seminar. The seminar was beneficial because it made clear that administration is not always best qualified to make decisions on any given matter. In fact, those closest to the problem frequently have the best solution. We have proven this theory over and over in the many task forces that have worked on specific problems in recent months. Their efforts proved that input from a broad range of people leads to the best decisions.

Several weeks ago, many of us filled out questionnaires on our attitudes about the Clinic. The data from these questionnaires reveal a profile of where we stand and what some of our problems are.

Morale of physicians and employees is nowhere near ideal.

Considerable confusion exists about our mission and goals.

Considerable confusion also exists about the chain of command. Commonly, a person trying to get a solution to a problem will go to several other people in different positions, leading to wasted energy as well as frustration.

A tremendous lack of decisiveness results from no one's being clear on who has authority to do what. This lack of decisiveness runs through the entire organization, from the Board of Directors down to the supervisors.

Most employees aspire to quite high standards, and in some cases they expect more of themselves than those in leadership do. Occasionally, people make decisions more on the basis of what is good for the physicians than what is good for the employees or even for the patients.

Commonly, members of one group or department don't listen to other groups.

Too little cooperation exists between departments. When one division needs temporary help, too few individuals from other divisions volunteer. Protecting one's own division at the expense of another's erodes trust.

Even within the same department, one person is unwilling to assist another.

We lack a well-developed reward system. Too often, someone who does a job well doesn't receive even a pat on the back.

Even more often, we do not invoke sanctions for someone who is doing a mediocre job, just squeaking by.

We have no formal training program to develop leadership skills. We tend to promote people to supervisory positions without training them and allowing them to develop appropriate skills to handle their new roles.

We cannot easily or suddenly change the culture we have evolved. We will have to strengthen many links in the chain of command.

We are hiring a professional personnel manager who will assist not only in recruiting the highest-caliber personnel but also in training supervisors and in team building.

We will recruit a new Clinic manager . . . to help identify and handle many of the Clinic's everyday problems.

The Board of Directors is restructuring the entire administrative team and has appointed Dr. Fernandez to quarterback the team as Chief Executive Officer.

The Board will have a four-day retreat in late January to plan new projects the Clinic will be taking on.

The Board will also authorize new committees to handle the various tasks necessary to provide strong leadership in the Clinic.

The Board will ask employees to participate in more task forces to help deal with specific problems.

Our supervisors will take on new and greater responsibilities.

In short, we will ask all in the organization to elevate their standards of performance. Together, we can push one another to move the Clinic forward.

None of these changes will be easy, simple, or quick. Some of them will be hard for some people to accept. Many of us have grown comfortable in our current roles and would rather not strive for higher levels of performance. However, with the commitment that so many physicians and employees have already shown, we can't fail. Too many people have already invested significant energy in these changes. We have a lot of smart, dedicated people committed to this project. They have been willing to look at our weaknesses and to make plans to correct them. We have allowed several outside consultants to come in and analyze us. Our leadership is strongly committed to this project and has resolved not to let it fizzle, even when the going gets tough. A new, shared sense of our commitment to be the pre-eminent health-care organization in this region will be our motivation. This shared sense of mission will convert us from a loosely associated group of individual practitioners into a real organization, in the grandest sense of the word.

Editor's note: Sixteen of the physicians and non-physicians involved in the planning retreat wrote evaluations. Their comments were uniformly positive and optimistic.

CHART ENTRY

Memo to:	**All Staff**
From:	**CEO**
Date:	**January 27, 1985**
Subject:	**Report of Long-Range Planning Retreat**

The executive team participated in a long-range planning retreat January 24–27 at Black Mountain. Mr. Bruce Fritch coordinated this planning work. In the past, some of the Clinic's policies and decisions have been reactions to problems. In recent months, sentiment has been building for active decision-making that would anticipate, even avoid, problems. Only when we understand the big picture of where the Clinic wants to go can we align individual decisions with our goals.

The attached "Mission Statement of the Nalle Clinic" sets forth the Clinic's objectives. Please notice the commitment to providing high-quality patient-care through a team approach. By uniting us in this common effort, our mission will provide us many advantages, not the least of which is a more rewarding work environment. To achieve this goal, all of us must have the same vision of what we want our new Clinic to be.

We thoroughly analyzed both the strengths and the weaknesses of the various areas of the Clinic and concluded that nineteen separate areas need specific plans for improvement. These include financial management, growth, administrative systems, marketing, community participation, human-resource development, and performance measurement and assessment.

In the next several days, we will appoint members to each of the twelve priority task forces created. We will appoint and train team leaders and educate teams about their specific roles as well as how they fit into the larger perspective of the Clinic's planning and decision making. They will receive support in the form of the personnel or finances necessary to accomplish their specific tasks. They will report their activities and recommendations to the Board of Directors and, ultimately, to all personnel of the Clinic. The Board will also provide coordinators to increase the efficiency of the work of these groups. We will establish specific schedules for completing these actions. The Board will also continue its long-range planning.

This approach is a distinct departure from past methods of making decisions about problems. The quality of our decisions should improve dramatically. The result of this effort should be a more integrated clinic where all personnel will more clearly comprehend their roles in the organization and will, therefore, be able to make more significant contributions. Every role is critical to the success of the organization.

Past efforts like this in the Nalle Clinic and in other organizations have proven that these endeavors are worth the effort. The Board hopes that its commitment to improving the Clinic will flow down to all levels of the Clinic. If we can all pick up their enthusiasm, the Nalle Clinic's stature will skyrocket. Working in a clinic whose goal is to become the pre-eminent health-care facility in this region of the country will actually be fun. Our pride should be sufficient reward for the time, money, and energy the Clinic is committing.

The Board has set up a framework for success. In a short time, specific fruits of this labor should become apparent. When we ask you to make your contribution, please remember that your participation is essential to the overall success of our mission.

CHART ENTRY:
MISSION STATEMENT OF THE NALLE CLINIC

*T*he Nalle Clinic will provide to our patients comprehensive health care of the highest quality. In this cause, our organizational structure will give maximum support to our personnel.

We pledge that we will use our energies and talents to provide medical care that is compassionate and personal, cost efficient and convenient. In addition, we will offer innovative services and health-care programs.

We will recruit only the finest, most-qualified staff; conduct clinical research; commit to broad-based involvement in quality assessment; and encourage an effective education program for physicians, staff, patients, and community.

We dedicate ourselves to visionary leadership in medical and business practices, being ever mindful of our commitment to the unique individuals who constitute the Nalle Clinic. We will nurture their growth and pride in the organization.

We will preserve and enhance the integrity of the Clinic and will strive to be a source of comfort and support to the community.

By direction of the Board of Directors
January 27, 1985

CHART ENTRY:
LETTER TO IRV RUBIN

by Raymond Fernandez, M.D.
February 1, 1985

*D*ear Irv,

I have included a copy of our Mission Statement as well as a report to all of our personnel about the success of the long-range planning effort. Bruce Fritch's leadership of the Board in this effort was masterful. I was also tickled with the tremendous energy and commitment the Board exhibited in approaching this task.

I sense an understanding that "things are happening" permeating our organization, and a growing commitment to those things. It's not all easy, and some people are standing back in disbelief and with a challenging attitude. With time and patience, I think we will win their support.

Wouldn't it be wonderful if everyone in our organization could pick up some of the understanding that I obtained from your course? . . . I hope that Bruce will be able to do the same type of job here at the Clinic. I will certainly support him in that effort, and I encourage you to help walk him through the steps necessary to get to that position.

COMMENTARY: ORGANIZATIONAL CULTURE CHANGE: A SELF-HELP PROGRAM

by Irwin Rubin, Ph.D.

What is essential to quality patient care? Active commitment to, and full participation in, healing. As physician-CEO, Dr. Fernandez is dedicated to the Nalle Clinic. Though the patient has lots of different ideas and concerns, he keeps lines of communication open. He provides forums, structures, information, and communication skills. In so doing, he adapts and replicates a process used regularly by physicians in dealing with patients: the Weed process.

Quality care requires freedom of choice, commitment, full participation, and valid data, both subjective and objective. As the attending physician for the Nalle Clinic, Dr. Fernandez begins by interviewing his patient (December 13, 1984, memo). Together they make a thorough diagnosis of the Clinic's current state of health. Anonymous questionnaires are supplemented by publicly aired beliefs, pains, and anxieties. Through Dr. Fernandez's leadership, the patient begins taking personal responsibility for its own wellness. Influential parts of the patient are beginning to take action to heal themselves.

Individual patients take responsibility for their own wellness by having periodic medical check-ups, including X-ray diagnoses of the functioning and health of vital internal organs. Similarly, health-care organizations intent on growing up, regardless of their stage of development, will begin by diagnosing their climate. For Stage-III organizations, such X-ray diagnoses are matters of regularly scheduled organizational health maintenance.

An organization's climate, the working atmosphere that prevails within the organization, has proven to be a strong indicator of the organization's health and performance. All of us respond to our environment. If we are uncomfortable in particular surroundings, we focus on that discomfort and use our energy to deal with the circumstances creating it. In a win-win organizational climate, individuals cooperate in striving for their common goal: excellence in patient-centered quality care.

The anonymous questionnaire and open-group discussion that Dr. Fernandez refers to in his December 13, 1984, memo reflect such an X-ray diagnosis of his patient's health. This diagnosis contains few surprises.[10] The process used, however, brings unrecorded hallway and coffee-room conversations into the open and

---

[10] See pp. 26–28.

increases people's commitment to take action. What follows will give you a taste of the process and a glimpse of the issues and insights such a diagnosis can provide. We'll highlight general qualitative patterns and themes, not detailed specific quantitative results.

Selecting a Sample

The purpose for doing the survey and the context within which the results are to be used determine the depth and breadth of the sample taken. An overview, akin to a total body scan, would be a typical first step. Any shadow areas uncovered would warrant follow-up diagnosis: focusing the camera's lens on a particular part of the body.

The Board of the Nalle Clinic convened the December 13, 1984, retreat. Their purpose was to consider changes that could profoundly impact the Clinic. To make and implement big decisions without at least taking the pulse of the organization would have been irresponsible patient care.

The pulse took the form of a climate survey, which 47 people responded to: influential physicians (28), including the entire Board and other formal and informal physician leaders; the most senior non-physician administrators (13), and a small number (6) of key technical support personnel (laboratory, X-ray technicians, and nursing supervisors). Those who completed the survey were invited to attend the retreat so they could share their own feelings and experiences. They put meat on the bones of the anonymous survey.

Format of the Survey

The survey instrument focused on an inventory of specific behaviors known to be characteristic of organizations in search of excellence. The questionnaire measured several dimensions,[11] including *responsibility* (the extent to which individuals are accountable for their own job performance), *excellence* (the extent to which individuals are committed to producing quality work), and *team spirit* (the extent to which individuals support one another personally and professionally).

The respondents were asked to share their perceptions about the specific behaviors from three perspectives:

(A) Awareness of Importance

An organization's values are the core—the heart and soul—of its climate. The first perspective focused upon the extent of people's cognitive awareness of the

---

[11] The current version of the climate survey measures 7 dimensions via 84 quantitative and 5 qualitative questionnaire items.

importance of each behavior to the achievement of organizational excellence. In excellence-oriented climates people agree on what it takes to deliver quality patient-centered care.

(B) Behavioral Frequency

In a win-win organization, management leads by example, aligning its own behavior with organizational values. The second perspective focused upon the frequency of each behavior in people's day-to-day experience. Excellence-oriented climates strive to "walk their talk," to minimize discrepancies between what they say and what they do.

(C) Consequences of Occurrence

Continuous learning from experience is key to the search for excellence. Without constant feedback and encouragement, learning from experience cannot take place. The third perspective focused upon the consequences–formal and/or informal–that would be expected by persons if, and when, they exhibited each of the behaviors.

The quantitative scales used are reproduced below.

(A) Awareness of Importance

You are being asked for your personal perception or belief about the extent to which the behavior would be expected to contribute to organizational excellence at the Nalle Clinic. (Ignore, on this scale, whether or not you perceive the behavior to exist at the Nalle Clinic.)

1	2	3	4	5	6	7
Major Hindrance			Neutral			Critical Positive Impact
This behavior cannot help us at all in achieving excellence			No impact one way or another			Without this behavior, achieving excellence will be doubtful

(B) Behavioral Frequency

Next, review the same item of behavior from the perspective of the extent to which, in your personal experience, you see each behavior reflected at the Nalle Clinic. (Ignore, on this scale, any beliefs you may have about the importance of the behavior in producing excellence or the consequences of the behavior.)

1	2	3	4	5	6	7
I hardly ever see any indications of this behavior being exhibited			I see indications of this behavior exhibited on somewhat frequent basis			I see indications of this behavior exhibited almost on a daily basis

(C) Consequences of Occurrence

Next, review the same item of behavior from the perspective of <u>your percep-tion</u> of the consequences—formal and/or informal—which would be expect-ed by the person(s) who exhibit(s) the behavior.

1	2	3	4	5	6	7
This behavior would be discouraged			This behavior would receive no clear encouragement or discouragement			This behavior would be clearly encouraged

Feeding Back the Survey Results

Several anonymous feedback summaries were prepared. Each focused on a dif-ferent facet of the X-ray. Subgroup summaries allowed a comparison of how differ-ent groups experienced the climate, for example, non-physician administrators and the physician Board. By examining the variance in perceptions (as distinct from the mean scores), among the members of a specific subgroup, inferences could be made as to the tightness versus looseness of various subcultures. For example, a depart-ment whose members pooled and shared equally all income could be expected, over time, to develop a highly consensual picture of the climate in their department. Regardless of the mean score on any particular climate dimension, this subsample could be expected to reflect high agreement (low variance). In contrast, a depart-ment whose members, for whatever reasons, were more loosely connected might reflect wider variances in perceptions.

I do not imply that tightness is better than looseness. Perceptual similarities may minimize conflicts and increase the possibility of group think. On the other hand, a diversity of perspectives can add richness and creativity as long as a common mis-sion provides focus. Conducting surveys and discussing their results provides a valuable opportunity to manage the organization's climate.

Individuals kept copies of their own responses so they could compare their per-ceptions with the anonymous group summaries. Individuals were free to share their personal perceptions, and many chose to do so during small subgroup discussions. Such willingness and openness are important signs that the patient-organization is beginning to take responsibility for its own growth.

Reading the X-ray

The reading of an organizational climate survey, like reading a patient's X-ray, requires a delicate combination of science and art. Both are examined from many perspectives. Interpretation requires the active involvement of the human organism being diagnosed. Before treatment can begin, first impressions and intuitive hunch-es must be followed by deeper probing and more extensive diagnoses.

To acknowledge these realities and to ensure the patient's right to privacy, I will present and discuss only examples of surface-level, overall patterns (N=47).

This sample of key individuals was very aware of (average mean scores almost a perfect 7), and in very high agreement about (low standard deviations), the importance of the following example behavioral patterns:

- setting high, but achievable, goals
- taking time to praise people when they did something well
- trusting people to do their jobs (versus watching over their shoulders all the time)
- looking for the cause of a problem when a mistake was made and learning from it (versus seeking to place the blame on a person).

At the other end of the scale, there was a typical lower mean score (slightly over 4) and high level of disagreement (standard deviation in excess of 1.5) on the issue of "exceeding the limits of one's formal authority when necessary to get the job done." As would be expected of an organization in Stage I, a fraternity stage of development, the Board (physician-keepers of the brotherhood) and the non-physician administrators were at opposite ends of this bell-shaped curve.

Commandments from on high may be set in stone, but life in the trenches requires trust and flexibility. The formal organization will specify the job to be done, and then the informal organization will determine how it actually gets done. Ironically, as a board member, a physician might agree to certain behavior guidelines, but as a practitioner, exceed these limits. This inconsistency, born of privileged status, frustrates non-physician administrators.

By and large, the values that the Nalle Clinic agreed were important to the achievement of excellence indicated a healthy heart and soul. The patient-organization, from my own experience, reflected a healthy level of conscious awareness.

Their *normal* developmental challenge—and I cannot stress enough their normality as a Stage-I organization—was to bring their day-to-day behavior into alignment with their conscious awareness of important values. The search for excellence is a never-ending journey, a process. Each plateau of achievement merely provides the sanctuary for a brief rest and the opportunity to learn from past experience.

On the basis of this assessment, Dr. Fernandez activates immediate, short-term therapies: he brings new blood on board. He authorizes new committees to focus healing energies on "the various tasks necessary to provide strong leadership in the Clinic." The patient and the provider collaborate to determine these tasks. Dr. Fernandez appropriately emphasizes the vision of a healthier future as well as the absence of guarantees and quick fixes.

It is important to emphasize that the map is not the territory. A climate survey, like an X-ray, can only suggest areas needing attention. Formal reward systems, clear value-driven mission statements, simple structures, informal pats on the back, heavy investments in training and development—these are ingredients essential for the creation of excellence-oriented organizational climates. All of these ingredients are necessary.

The organization is a patient whose chief complaint and presenting illness reflect normal growing pains. It wanted to grow beyond its childhood (condominium) orientation. As its leader, Dr. Fernandez reports in his December 13, 1984, chart entry that senior management had demonstrated its verbal commitment to organizational cultural change. This chart entry itself is one example of how senior management dealt with individuals in the Clinic: management provided information about what the organizational cultural change might involve and gave people the freedom to choose to go through the process. Both physicians and non-physicians in senior management had already freely committed themselves to the cultural change, and in the final section of the December 13, 1984, memo, many of them enthusiastically stated their reasons.

This memo also serves as a new social contract, announcing to the Clinic that from now on, senior management's behavior will be different and that it will serve as the example for the rest of the Clinic to follow:

> The Board of Directors is restructuring the entire administrative team and has appointed a new chief executive officer. . . . The Board will also authorize new committees to handle the various tasks necessary to provide strong leadership in the Clinic. . . . The Board will ask employees to participate in more task forces to help deal with specific problems. Our supervisors will take on new and greater responsibilities. . . . We will ask all in the organization to elevate their standards of performance. Together, we can push one another to move the Clinic forward.

Anonymous questionnaires have described the realities that members of the Clinic observe and the ideals they desire. Senior management has accepted responsibility for the dissatisfactions the questionnaires revealed. The questionnaires also revealed readiness, motivation, and ability to change. As the memo stated, "Most employees aspire to quite high standards, and in some cases they expect more of themselves than those in leadership do."

Dr. Fernandez closes the body of this memo by reiterating senior management's commitment to organizational cultural change, to making the Clinic "the pre-eminent health-care organization in this region." Developmentally, I associate such a mission statement with a Stage-III organization in search of excellence. As I have noted, the operating psychological contract for such a Stage-III organization

is unique and very expensive. The organization provides security from arbitrary layoffs, but not from dismissal for continued unacceptable perfor-mance. It also provides regular opportunities for challenge, autonomy, and synergy. In return, individual members are expected to give up a piece of their *souls*—to invest of their *selves* in the business.

Once we've made a painful decision, we have a natural tendency to hope, if not act as though, we can detour around, or speed up, the steps the decision requires. Although its mission statement points to Stage III, the Nalle Clinic (and others like it) cannot avoid going through Stage II, which provides the training ground, the toughening up, necessary to move to Stage III.

Continuing his practice of organizational healing, Dr. Fernandez begins his January 27, 1985, chart entry with updates to the patient: he describes actions he committed management to at the close of the December 13, 1984, retreat. Both open-ness of information—central to informed consent—and reliability in meeting com-mitments—central to developing trust—are essential to a successful doctor-patient relationship. Senior management commits to taking concrete action to support cul-tural change: beyond their written mission statement, they promise to provide lead-ership, training, and money to those who will plan for and implement the cultural change. Dr. Fernandez makes careful and extensive use of teams–task-force cells–as skeletal reinforcements to stabilize a human organism struggling to maintain its bal-ance in the face of intense but normal growing pains. He mobilizes twelve such ad-hoc committees to treat the nineteen separate areas that need improvement.

Growing up, Dr. Fernandez notes, will require an approach to management that is "a distinct departure from past methods of making decisions about problems. The quality of our decisions should improve dramatically. The result of this effort should be a more integrated clinic where all personnel will more clearly comprehend their roles in the organization and will, therefore, be able to make more significant con-tributions."

Organizationally, growing up means all parts of the body must take a larger share of personal responsibility to keep the entire organization strong. "Every role is crit-ical to the success of the organization." Dr. Fernandez informs the patient once again that its full "participation is essential to the overall success of our mission."

The words *every role is critical* and *our mission* are vital to leadership in organiza-tional cultural change. The mission statement is the entire Nalle Clinic's, by direc-tion of the Board of Directors; yet it is individuals who act as leaders. Whether or not these initiatives are mutually beneficial, and at what costs to whom, depend on the quality of the exchange. The quality of the partnership, the relationship between a patient and a provider, determines the outcome of healing.

Creating the necessary win-win results depends on strong interpersonal skills, courage, and persistence. The preceding memos allow us to analyze Dr. Fernandez's style of communication, *how* he communicates what he says he is going to do, and what the patient needs to do. A physician-CEO's style of communication is crucial to influencing the patient-organization to fulfill its part of the leadership transaction.

There are many useful programs for developing communication skills. The model I use is from my course *The ABCs of Win-Win Relationships*. In all of our human interactions, we use our energies either to *push* thoughts, feelings, or ideas toward someone or to *pull* thoughts, feelings, or ideas from someone. When we *push* to shape and direct others' thinking and behaviors, we can use four styles: focusing on facts and logic, we *describe* what has happened in the past or is happening at the moment, and we *prescribe* what could or should happen in the future; focusing on our feelings, we *appreciate* the significance and value of what has happened in the past or is happening at the moment, and we *inspire* others to work together to achieve common goals.

When we *pull* from others, we also use four styles. Our first responsibility is to *attend,* to make sure we are receptive to what others *push.* Whether we agree or disagree with what others *push,* when we *ask* for their thoughts, feelings, or ideas, we must keep an open mind. We use a variety of verbal and non-verbal cues to communicate that we *understand* others' thoughts and ideas. When we sense and acknowledge others' feelings, we *empathize.*

These samples of his public communiques demonstrate a balanced push-pull pattern.

Let us look more closely at Dr. Fernandez's December 13, 1984, memo. After clearly and candidly *describing* what happened at the first retreat (including the dirty laundry), Dr. Fernandez *prescribes* the future implications: "In short, we will ask all in the organization to elevate their standards of performance." He immediately follows this new expectation with an *inspirational* reminder of the power of teamwork: "Together we can push one another to move the Clinic forward."

Such a tall order is bound to stir up anxiety, resistance, and cynicism. Dr. Fernandez then shifts to communicating an understanding of, and *empathy* with, his patient: "None of these changes will be easy, simple, or quick. Some of them will be hard for some people to accept. Many of us have grown comfortable in our current roles and would rather not strive for higher levels of performance."

While not denying the validity of these feelings, Dr. Fernandez is careful to *appreciate* past achievements and current strengths: "However, with the commitment that so many physicians and employees have already shown," the "many smart, dedicated people committed to the project will not," he *prescribes,* "let it fizzle." He follows with further *inspiration:* "A new, shared sense of our commitment to be the preeminent health-care organization in this region will be our motivation. This shared sense of mission will convert us from a loosely associated group of individual practitioners into a real organization, in the grandest sense of the word."

Not everyone will agree with Dr. Fernandez's vision. He *asks* his patient to seek second and third opinions and to keep an open mind: "We invite you to contact any of these people [retreat attendees who publicly aired their own feelings along with Dr. Fernandez] and solicit their further comments."

Dr. Fernandez uses the tools of persistence: *descriptive* data, *prescriptive* recommendations, *appreciative* judgments, and *inspired* visions. He's equally determined to honorably discharge his persistent responsibilities, to stay in close, human touch with his patient. He remains patiently *attentive, asks* for counsel, expresses *understanding* of diverse concerns, and demonstrates *empathy.*

Leadership in organizational culture change, as previously noted, requires the flexible and humane application, based upon valid diagnoses, of generic healing therapies. Quick-fix formulas will not result in permanent healing. Each treatment plan must be tailored to the specific and evolving needs of the patient-organization. My commentary on the initial treatment plan developed by Dr. Fernandez and the Nalle Clinic will, therefore, take the form of a series of questions. These questions will serve as a checklist of issues to be addressed by physician-CEO's and their patient organizations to determine their readiness, motivation, and ability to journey in search of excellence.

1. Mission question: "Has the creation of the required agreed-upon mission statement been the result of an extensive group process?"

Many organizations begin to sink themselves by avoiding the very painful and time-consuming requirement to agree together on "where we are going." They delegate this responsibility to one (their physician-CEO) or to a small handful of individuals.

The irony of this trap is that the quality of the resulting statement, in terms of the words on paper, may be identical to that which might result from an expensive and gut-wrenching process among a broadly based group. Since the quality of the process is as important as the final content, skipping the process guarantees two potential deadly outcomes, both related to commitment. Let's look at these one at a time.

The first potential problem is the lack of psychological ownership of change. The famous Western Electric "Hawthorne effect" experiments verified what our common sense always knew: when you want to make a change, you have to involve the people who will be changing. Let them help plan and implement the ideas. The same principle applies to the Nalle Clinic: involve the physician-CEO, the Board of Directors, and the senior executives. Put them in a room and let them hash out a mission statement together. Then the words of the mission statement can come to life because many people agree on them and want them to succeed.

The second potential problem is the lack of continuity of change. Another advantage of having several people work on the mission statement is that they are less likely to make inappropriate, and potentially dangerous, wholesale changes: to throw out the baby with the bath water. Past successes, like a child's favorite toy, can ease the pain of moving to a new plateau of excellence. Many treasured and essential learnings occurred as an organization arrived at its current state of development. Some pieces of its proud history will be critical to keep on board as its new journey begins.

2. Structure question: "Have temporary life-support structures been established to help people cope with the early stages of transition?"

The growing-up process requires us to release familiar, old patterns and to face new challenges. Like a patient who has just endured open-heart surgery, an organization embarking on a journey toward wellness will need temporary structures to ease the transition, particularly because it's traveling into uncharted territory.

The organization's vital signs must be checked frequently. Management by walking around and regular, loosely structured group meetings are the keys to checking its pulse. Managers will know how everyone's doing, how everyone's handling the normal and expected anxiety in times of change. Holding the patient's hand also ensures that complications can be diagnosed and treated early.

These will not be easy steps to take. Human nature being what it is, those seen as responsible for the patient-organization's stress and anxiety will not always be greeted with open arms. It will be tempting for them to stay in the office, hiding behind mountains of paperwork, in order to avoid hostility. But it's essential to stay in touch.

3. Procedures question: "Are enough tools available to ensure that individuals are ready, willing, and able to support the mission?"

Most organizations *severely underestimate* what is required to support behavioral changes during major transitions. People must develop new habits and unlearn some old ones. They must develop teamwork.

A Stage-I organization is like a baseball team. While some players may be gifted enough to play more than one position—shortstop and second base, for example—most players specialize. Baseball's fundamental nature is low, on-line interdependence. Except for the occasional fly ball, it takes pairs (pitcher and catcher) or trios (infielder, first baseman, and catcher, as a backup) to play the game: to throw and catch and tag the runner out.

A Stage-II organization is more like a football team. The quarterback calls the play, and *in theory*, it will be successful *if* all eleven players perform their roles perfectly. Compared to baseball, football is characterized by higher levels of on-line interdependence. While players specialize, they need other skills, too: a tackle might also intercept the ball and run for a touchdown. A Yankees player who tries out for the Miami Dolphins will need dramatically different teamwork muscles. The Bo

Jacksons of the world are rare.

Finally, a Stage-III organization is like a basketball team, which uses very few pre-set plays. While skilled players are necessary, teamwork is even more important in this highly interdependent game. Teamwork means practicing together under game conditions long enough and hard enough to be able, as Bill Russell once commented, to see the play developing "in slow motion" and know "intuitively" where a teammate will be in the next split second.

While numbers are impossible to specify, it is safe to say that an organization can *not* earmark too much time and money for training budgets. Before pushing off on its journey into uncharted waters, an organization must stash skilled training resources on board.

4. The question of intangibles: "Do you have faith in your mission and belief in yourself?"

The last factor on the treatment-plan checklist will ultimately determine the journey's success or failure; yet it will be impossible to assess before the fact. Just as medicine can bring unprecedented knowledge, skill, and technology to a patient's care, it is often the patient's spiritual will to live that tips the scales of the healing process. Similarly, other people and events—a family intervention or a car crash—might bring an alcoholic into A.A., but the program of growing up will succeed only if the alcoholic accepts an underlying faith in a higher-order God and believes, heart and soul, that he or she is doing God's will.

As health-care organizations and their physician leaders move through their stages of development, their underlying reasons for embarking on these journeys will be severely tested and retested. This will be particularly true of those who dare to venture out of Stage II and make the quantum leap required to sail to a new world. Those who are successful will be driven by a belief that excellence in patient-centered care will be best delivered by self-actualizing organizations. Organizational culture change—the continuous process of growing up—is fundamentally a self-help, self-healing program.

In closing his February 1, 1985, chart entry, Dr. Fernandez expresses cautious optimism concerning the success of the self-help relationship between himself and his patient, the Nalle Clinic: "I sense an understanding that things are happening . . . . I think we will win their support."

Physician leaders, like Dr. Fernandez, will experience dramatic transformations in their self-images. They will have to surrender their deeply ingrained roles as the primary providers of quality care in patient treatment. In its place they will have to "grow up," to treat entire organizations of providers as patients in need of quality care. Such transformational journeys will trigger predictable psychological and behavioral dynamics.

In Part Three, we move from February 1, 1985, to December 5, 1988. During that period, Dr. Fernandez and I met a dozen times and spoke by phone many more times. Many of our conversations had to do with quality care and leadership, and the differences, if any, between the two. During one conversation, I asked Dr. Fernandez to describe the feelings of being CEO of an organization evolving out of its medical-condominium orientation.

What follows is Dr. Fernandez's account of how leading such a mission feels. He gives us his personal perspective on the process of leadership and organizational cultural change, almost four years to the day since he formally accepted the role as chief provider of the care team responsible for the Nalle Clinic.

Part Three:

Progress Report

DR. RAYMOND FERNANDEZ'S PERSONAL CHART ENTRY:

Edited Transcript of an Audiotape Sent to Irv Rubin
December 5, 1988

*I*n making the transition from physician to medical director and CEO, I crossed the invisible line between being us and being *them*. I remain sensitive to this distinction, and others cite it when it seems to serve their purposes. No matter how hard the physicians try to cover up their feelings, to them I am clearly a traitor. Understanding the psychodynamics of the situation does not ease the pain of having one of my close colleagues reject me because of my new role.

Although I had no difficulty logically seeing the need to give up my established practice, with which I had become very comfortable, announcing and making the necessary split was not easy to do. Telling my patients and my peers that I had decided to leave them was emotionally trying, particularly with members in my call group. They considered me disloyal, a traitor, because their lives would immediately become more difficult: they would have to tighten their belts to take more nights on call. Their career plans were entwined with mine, and now I had unilaterally decided to desert them. The way I felt I needed to behave for the greater good of the organization would, I know, leave some feeling that I had put other interests ahead of theirs. Thus, they became intent on discouraging me from carrying out my intentions.

Initially, I tried to strike a compromise by keeping one foot in my practice and one in administration. I even tried maintaining the old call schedule for a while. But before long, I realized that this compromise was not workable. I was being unfair to my family, my patients, my peers, and myself. I would have to leave behind the financial and emotional security I had built over several years in my practice.

One doesn't usually leave one comfortable situation for another situation unless the second one seems quite clearly dependable. In my case, I could not depend on my peers to support my decision to move to administration. I had no role models there to welcome me or serve as advisors. The only advice I was getting from those I had grown to trust was not to make the change. To convince myself that those around me didn't understand the situation well enough to give me good long-term advice, that I would have to make my decision without any encouragement, forced me to perceive myself in the role of a crusader. I was willing to sacrifice myself and my happiness to do something for my peers that they couldn't yet see was good for them, but that they would eventually appreciate. The situation was analogous to recommending a blood transfusion to a Jehovah's Witness. We know from our training and experience that the advice is good; we know that the patient is not able to accept that advice; but we feel we've got to give the advice anyway.

Realizing that I had no formal training in business, leadership, management, or organizational psychology heightened my personal insecurity. The search committee were unable to give me a clear definition of the role they were asking me to assume. In fact, after they selected me, they asked me to write the original job description. They also asked me where I was going to get some management experience.

At this stage, I had to develop courage. With very little in the way of guidelines or advisors, I had to have the courage to make my own decisions about what was best for me and for the organization. With no guidelines for measuring success or predicting the long-term consequences my decisions would have on me and the group, I had a strong fear of failure. And I recalled a lesson I had learned years earlier, when I first hypnotized my college roommate.

I had read a couple of books on hypnosis and had talked about it with my father, who used it in his medical practice. I felt that I had a pretty good grasp of the didactic basis for hypnotism. I presented myself to my roommate as "having a lot of experience." He wouldn't stop begging me to put him into a trance that would allow him to stop smoking and to study harder without distractions. When I finally agreed to hypnotize him, the ease with which I put him into a trance amazed me. And terrified me. What if I couldn't awaken him? What if I caused this poor fellow some type of harm? Why had I allowed myself even to try such a thing? Somehow I bluffed my way through and got him out of the trance. But the realization of the responsibility that went along with that mysterious power remains a frightening, valuable lesson for me.

At this stage, I also had to learn to deal with isolation. In this organizational culture that had not had someone in a role of power and authority, physicians have trouble communicating with me. Their view of me as a traitor has shut off certain channels. They neither understand nor appreciate my new role, although they apparently sense that it is essential. I have a related problem with some of the administrators, because as CEO, I am now their boss. They, too, think a physician in an administrative role is a waste: administrators should administer, and physicians should treat patients. With no real peer group, I don't feel that I can let down my guard with anyone. While both groups clearly want me to succeed, they need to see me fail to prove their belief that physicians don't make good administrators.

I ask myself, "Can I do this job? Do I want this job?" I have the luxury of being able to go back to being a physician. On days when the aggravation becomes extreme, I remember how easy my job was when all I had to do was make simple life-and-death decisions for individual patients. But I remind myself that as a physician, I had to put my patient's needs before my own desires. Now, I have this same feeling of obligation to the organization: my patient needs me.

However, the manager's role has significant differences. I don't see the results of a decision until some time after I've made it. Frequently, my colleagues ask me to tell them what they need to do, which sometimes translates into my telling them how to conduct their practice, but which they see as my telling them how to treat patients. This sort of conflict is ongoing. The frustration it creates seems pervasive, since most of the highly intelligent professionals I work with have little appreciation for the big picture I must see. They look only at their individual practices and their individual realities. One of my most important duties is to translate and communicate others' ideas. However, listeners tend to mistrust a translator they must depend on.

Rejection from my peers is painful. They seem to enjoy disagreeing openly with decisions I make. Disagreement with an individual decision tends to lead to loss of confidence in the competence and authority of my position. Any decision I make is bound to irritate at least ten percent of my constituents. However, no two decisions irritate the same ten percent, so by the time I have made ten decisions, I have irritated everyone. The fact that these peers are my equals in the medical culture makes functioning as the decision maker that much harder. I have difficulty accepting that I must accept ultimate blame for all failures in the organization. So I constantly wonder if it's really worth it. Like the physician who has lost a patient or become embroiled in a lawsuit, I wonder if the anger and frustration I feel are worth the reward.

Organized medicine faces many challenges: do we need to circle the wagons, fight, give in, or learn to make friends with the new system? In the midst of this indecision, organizations ask the physician-manager to lead the troops down the right path. We see groups in our community succeeding in joint ventures with hospitals, while other groups ask us to lead the fight against "those damned hospital administrators." In the role of physician-executive, we are supposed to have a clear vision of what is best for our organizations and where to lead them. The simple truth is that we really don't know. Yet to keep our positions as effective leaders, we've got to keep telling our troops where we are taking them.

The other side of the story is that what I am doing now is fun. Having the power and autonomy of a decision maker is something to which I think most physicians naturally aspire. The highs are higher and the lows, lower in my current position than in medical practice. As patients literally put their lives in their physician's hands, so, too, the life of the organization is in mine. The challenge of controlling a complex organization's culture, financial performance, quality control, and morale is exciting. As the organization progresses through change and growth, I take a parent's pride in its successes. Still, the fear and frustration of dealing with the unknown is something physician-managers have to live with every day. Like Columbus, we have to realize that most of the people actually hope we'll fall off the end of the world so that they can remain secure in their belief that the world is flat.

COMMENTARY: LEADING BY EXAMPLE

by Irwin Rubin, Ph.D.

*I*n many ways the Nalle Clinic did not want to be led. Here the patient, not an individual but a collection of providers, rejects Dr. Fernandez. The birth of an extended self-image, one that admits collections of providers as one's patients, triggers deep, emotional reactions. We see Dr. Fernandez's hopes and fears in his December 1988 chart entry. "I am clearly a traitor," Dr. Fernandez says; yet he has no trouble understanding that the rejections are not personal. He is able to control the pain rather than avoid it.

Reacting to the imminent death of a part of his old self-image, his psyche begins to negotiate a series of devil's bargains. "Initially," Dr. Fernandez says, "I tried to strike a compromise by keeping one foot in my practice and one in administration." For someone of his integrity, such a compromise will be short lived. He quickly realizes that this compromise is "unfair to my family, my patients, my peers, and myself."

Dr. Fernandez is caught between reference groups ("between being us and being *them*") and between self-images ("I am clearly a traitor"), without "financial and emotional security," without even the potential security of "a clear definition of the role [the search committee] were asking me to assume," and with peers "intent on discouraging me from carrying out my intentions." The intensity of these conflicting emotions calls for a more intense devil's bargain. When rational compromise does not work, psychological compromise becomes tempting. Trying such a compromise "in the role of a crusader . . . willing to sacrifice myself and my happiness . . . was analogous," Dr. Fernandez said, "to recommending a blood transfusion to a Jehovah's Witness." And with similar consequences.

By confronting and accepting what began as a "strong fear of failure," Dr. Fernandez uncovers an equally strong fear of success. Through a process Jung calls synchronicity, Dr. Fernandez recalls a lesson in humility from many years earlier, which began with his success in hypnotizing a friend: "The ease with which I put him into a trance amazed me. And terrified me. What if I couldn't awaken him? [What if he died?] What if I caused this poor fellow [this entire organization-as-patient] some type of harm?" As life and death are equal parts of the experience, so are healing and failing.

Psychic acceptance of aloneness and impermanence are keys to personal succession. (*Succession*, as I use the term here, is "the process of moving from one stage of development to another.") Paradoxically, increased openness and acceptance are the best defense against peers who consider Dr. Fernandez a traitor. "I also had to learn to deal with isolation. . . . While both groups clearly want me to succeed, they need to see me fail to prove their belief that physicians don't make good administrators." Increasing comfort in the fact that both administrators and physicians know that "as CEO, I am now their boss" does not relieve Dr. Fernandez's isolation, the loneliness at the top: "With no real peer group, I don't feel that I can let down my guard with anyone."

Self-doubt creeps into Dr. Fernandez's thoughts: "Can I do this job? . . . But I remind myself that as a physician, I had to put my patient's needs before my own desires. Now, I have this same feeling of obligation to the organization: my patient needs me." A new self-image is taking hold. Dr. Fernandez has to act, fully aware that the consequences will be far-reaching, but seldom universally good or desirable: "By the time I have made ten decisions, I have irritated everyone."

Only a special breed of physician can make the transition to physician-executive. And only a special breed of person in that position will acknowledge that, "In the role of physician-executive, we are supposed to have a clear vision of what is best for our organizations and where to lead them. The simple truth is that we really don't know. Yet to keep our positions as effective leaders, we've got to keep telling our troops where we are taking them." I'm pleased, although not surprised, to see that for such a person, Ray Fernandez, "The other side of the story is that what I am doing now is fun."

In the memo of December 5, 1988, the ambivalent forces of human nature seemed to be in a state of peaceful coexistence—fear of success balancing the capacity to succeed, but only temporarily. Succession is a never-ending process. From the high points we can draw strength and insight, which we will need to climb the next mountain. Growth was causing some of the same symptoms Dr. Fernandez noted four years earlier to reappear, along with some new ones. Conflict within the Nalle Clinic over its control had become public record. The January 15, 1990, edition of the weekly *Business Journal* of Charlotte carried the headline "Nalle Lawsuit Vs. [a physician who left the Clinic to go out on his own, violating a contract he signed when he joined the Clinic] Heads to Appellate Court." The accompanying story stated, "The conflict with [the physician] isn't the first time Nalle has battled to enforce its restrictive covenant."

Five days later, the Charlotte *Observer* headlined, "Nalle Clinic Considers Taking on Financial Partner." According to the article, declining revenues, a result of the rapid growth and external environmental changes, led the patient to seek a new partner to "strengthen our financial position and assure our future." The report quoted Dr. Fernandez: "We had a bad third quarter. The fourth quarter was much improved. We need some capital. It's not a new need, and it's not an emergency need. It's not something we'd die without."

On March 1, 1990, the Nalle Clinic exercised its inalienable right to a second opinion. A process that had begun some five years earlier came to its own unique conclusion. Under Dr. Fernandez's leadership, the Nalle Clinic had taken the steps necessary to move away from its condominium roots and to become a more mature business organization. According to the March 5 Charlotte *Observer*, "Attempting to strengthen its finances and its future, the Nalle Clinic finalized a joint venture Thursday with PhyCor, a Nashville-based company that will manage the Clinic's business and provide money for expansion. . . . Under the agreement, [Dr.] Fernandez steps down as chief executive officer of the Clinic but remains medical director."

Knowledge without wisdom is useless. And wisdom is impossible without the courage to learn from experience. However hard we may try to control them, processes of human growth and development have a pace and a rhythm of their own. Part Four gives us a view of the human experience of death and dying as Dr. Fernandez struggles to accept the painful realization that he is about to become the first past-physician-CEO of the Nalle Clinic. His goal five years earlier was to assist his patient to grow into a more business-like organization. Unanticipated stresses caused the evolution to proceed at a pace that surprised everyone. Although this stage of development ended somewhat traumatically, Dr. Fernandez and his patient-organization have achieved the results they wanted. He has discharged his leadership responsibilities, and his patient has discharged him.

COMMENTARY:
REFLECTIONS OF A SEASONED VETERAN

by Henry Berman, M.D.
President and CEO of Group Health Northwest

T he history of the Nalle Clinic and of Dr. Raymond Fernandez's struggles as its first physician-CEO is one that many group practices and physician managers have experienced in the past decade. A number of changes in the environment have forced the profession to respond in ways that have led to experiences such as this one. These changes include an increasing number of physicians, more competition from other health-care providers, more pressure from the government and employers for cost-containment, higher expectations from patients, and a dramatic increase in the number of managed-care organizations.

As Dr. Fernandez described in his introduction, from its founding in 1921, the Clinic had grown to 40 physicians by 1975 and then doubled in size in less than 15 years. In response to environmental pressures, many group practices follow this pattern. It is a way of dealing with increased specialization and competition and demands for efficiency, and it enables the physicians to contract with HMO's and PPO's to protect or increase their patient base. However, many groups do not appreciate the importance of high-quality management in achieving their ambitious goals. For others, this appreciation is primarily intellectual until they hear the hard knocks of reality at their front doors. The Nalle Clinic was no exception.

We can trace this problem back to its roots in the Clinic's decision to make Dr. Fernandez its first medical director. In correspondence with me, Dr. Fernandez says his honest assessment of that decision in 1980 is that, of the three candidates for the position, "the organization found me to be the least threatening." Dr. Fernandez describes himself as having no prior experience with medical management. Someone with a bit of experience might have recognized that he was encountering a Groucho Marx paradox: Groucho turned down membership in a country club, refusing to belong to any club that would accept him as a member. My point is that, despite having no management experience, Dr. Fernandez was chosen for the job; and an organization that makes sure that it selects such a person is also going to make sure that that person cannot succeed.

Dr. Fernandez's correspondence with me also states that his "strongest skill was probably in being able to soothe troubled waters and look for areas of compromise rather than making dictatorial decisions." When group practices finally concede that they need a physician-manager, they typically choose a nice guy as their first medical director. Although strong interpersonal skills are necessary to be able to do this difficult job effectively, being too nice can be a liability.

We can find a useful analogy in styles of parenting. Authoritarian parents ("My way is the only way") eventually lose their ability to influence their children; authoritarian physician-CEO's fail much more quickly. Laissez-faire parents ("Do your own thing") are not very effective, but may well continue to have good interpersonal relationships with their children.[12] In my experience, laissez-faire physician-CEO's are not able to manage change in their organizations, yet this style is very popular. I believe that popularity may reflect the correct perception of how badly an authoritarian approach works out, coupled with a lack of understanding of what will work: the authoritative style. The authoritative style is not a compromise between the other two styles but a third, entirely different approach. Authoritative parents and leaders understand that they have knowledge and skills that are greater in certain areas, and responsibilities that they cannot shrug off. They also understand that wise leaders make most decisions after considerable consultation with those whom the decisions affect, that they hold as few decisions to themselves as possible, and that they encourage independent decision-making. Awareness of behavioral choices and their consequences plus the flexibility to respond to changing conditions are key. I do not believe that the Nalle Clinic was ready for an authoritative leader at that point in its history.

Another warning sign occurred when the Board "did not spell out the position's power and authority." The Clinic also lacked a formal goal-setting process and had never undertaken an evaluation of its leaders. In my experience, these shortcomings are also typical but a real danger to physician-executives. Our jobs are always complex, with many different groups to please, and, inevitably, displease. Setting goals flushes out the issues, and undergoing evaluation against those goals not only provides useful feedback to the physician-executive and the board but also protects the physician-executive against sudden shifts in the wind. Not having goals and an evaluation is similar to a physician's treating a patient with no plan and with no interest in measuring the success of the treatment.

On the other hand, as Irv Rubin points out, one real plus was the Clinic's realization that Dr. Fernandez would need training to be able to do his job effectively. Dr. Fernandez's ability to learn mainly from his mistakes is reassuring to the rest of us who have had the same experience. When I am very lucky, I learn from someone else's mistakes. More often, I learn from my own. Mediocre managers are not people who do not make mistakes, but those who do not learn from them. Experience is not the best teacher if no learning takes place.

The next key moment in this story occurred when Dr. Fernandez increased his

---

[12] *Editor's note:* A middle possibility exists here: reactive parents ("I'll do whatever makes you happy"), who quickly discover that their children do not know their own wants.

time to 85 percent administrative and went off call. "The Board readily agreed" to his suggestion, but others—in particular, those he shared call with—apparently did not. I don't know what process, if any, the Board used to make this decision, but they would have done well at this point to get buy-in from the entire physician group. I doubt that the statement "We all realized that my primary role had changed from being a clinician to being an administrator" is complete. Even though physicians in larger groups elect a board and supposedly delegate authority to that group, they seldom completely accept the fact that they have empowered that group to make certain decisions, usually those involving power or money or symbolically important issues. I have found no substitute for one-on-one or small-group discussions with the front-line physicians before making such decisions.

One such important symbolic issue is call. Sometimes it is a real issue as well, and the physicians left in the call schedule have to shoulder a heavy burden. But more often, that situation is not the problem, even when people act as if it is. They think, "Real doctors take call. Being a part-time administrator is all right, as long as you continue doing everything a real doctor does." Even though such an arrangement is neither sensible nor possible, physicians seem to be able to pretend that it is.

Starting without a firm foundation (the aforementioned Groucho Marx paradox) and moving forward into being an administrator without full support of the physicians left Dr. Fernandez in a precarious position in late 1984 when the Board asked him to become its first CEO. This was probably his last, best chance to clarify his authority, establish formal goals, develop an evaluation process, and put all these in writing in a formal contract.

One key phrase from the December 13, 1984, memo highlights the problem Dr. Fernandez faced: "The Board of Directors is restructuring the entire administrative team and has appointed Dr. Fernandez to quarterback the team as chief executive officer." The CEO should be the general manager or coach, not the quarterback. Even quarterbacks who call their own plays in the huddle—a rare and vanishing breed, to be sure—do so in the context of an overall game plan worked out by general management. The memo has already pointed out the fact that physicians caused many of the problems by making decisions that were good for them rather than good for the organization, as well as by protecting their own divisions at the expense of others'. These behaviors and attitudes, common in group practices, are among the most difficult issues to deal with effectively. The only hope a physician-manager has, to be able to make necessary changes, is to have the authority to make controversial decisions, not to be someone who just executes decisions others make.

The mission statement is worthy of discussion. Excellence-oriented, patient-centered mission statements are very much in vogue these days. The Nalle Clinic's rhetoric is impressive, but does it express what the physicians really wanted? Or did they want to be a more successful business, to have a better billing system and more capital, to earn more money? At this point, the Clinic is a classic Stage-I organization. Does it really want to leap to Stage III? Does it want to be a more successful Stage-I organization? Or does it want to move to Stage II? Aligning words and deeds is one of the leadership challenges.

Stage-I organizations are unable to deal with conflict in a healthy way. Instead of being impressed that those attending the January 1985 planning retreat specified nineteen separate areas in need of improvement, I would have been concerned that this might have represented pseudo-agreement, one way to avoid dealing with conflict. The group's coming up with nineteen areas for improvement makes me think of patients who see the light and agree to stop smoking and drinking and start exercising and dieting, all at the same time. Saying you will change everything ends up no different from deciding to change nothing. The most difficult task for a patient, or an organization, is to change *anything*. Coming up with a list of nineteen areas needing change is a first step. Choosing the priority need among them and making the change permanent is the giant step.

Landscape architects use the phrase "respect the genius of the place." They do not try to turn a desert home into a piece of England. The Clinic might have had better success trying to become the best Stage-I organization possible—and, in the process, starting inevitably on the path to Stage II, an effective business, rather than remaining a fraternity. Irv Rubin's commentary notes the organization's desire to skip the difficult process of going first to Stage II on the way to Stage III. I agree that thinking this jump is possible is an easy mistake to make since one wishes fervently that it were possible. It is no more possible than a child's becoming an adult without going through adolescence.

In Part Three, Dr. Fernandez provides unusual insight into how being a physician-executive feels. Because he wrote the notes a year before the most serious new developmental challenges became apparent, their insights are fresher than those we might develop in retrospect. Dealing with change means dealing with loss, and Elizabeth Kubler-Ross's model is useful in understanding the stages all of us go through when we experience change. For example, in dealing with the issue of giving up call, Dr. Fernandez experiences *denial* ("Everyone agreed that it was necessary"), *anger* ("They considered me a traitor"), *bargaining* ("I even tried maintaining the old call schedule for a while"), *sadness*, and *acceptance* ("I would have to leave behind the financial and emotional security I had built").

Dr. Fernandez's honesty in describing his isolation and fear of failure is unusual. Most of the time we are busy fooling others, no doubt in order to fool ourselves. Dr. Fernandez also expresses poignantly the loneliness of a CEO ("I could not depend on my peers. . . . I had no role models to welcome me. . . . The only advice I was getting . . . was not to make the change"). As lonely as being CEO is for anyone, it is even more difficult for physician-CEO's in their first such position. Non-physician

CEO's reach their positions after years of moving up an organization's ladder. Over the years, their peer group changes in a series of successive stages. As CEO's, their peers become CEO's they have come to know from similar organizations. But the physician-CEO must make the jump all at once, from a highly collegial relationship with dozens of physicians to a position with few, if any, role models, and no support systems. Like divers with no opportunity for decompression and re-acclimation, physician-CEO's find that too rapid a rise to the top can cause emotional disorientation and physical pain.

Dr. Fernandez's fear of failure is another common experience for physician-executives. By the time we have reached such a position, we have been involved in medicine for at least 15 years, often many more. We have a set of valuable skills that we can depend on, gratifying relationships with a large number of patients, a positive self-image, and the closest thing to a guaranteed ability to make a comfortable living that our society has to offer. Suddenly we find ourselves in a position with little or no training and little or no confidence in our skills, cut off from grateful patients and companionable colleagues, and at risk of being out of a job on short notice. Fear of failure represents a rational assessment of a difficult situation, not a panic response.

Dr. Fernandez also describes his difficulties gaining acceptance from the other administrators, who resented his being their leader despite, and perhaps because of, his apparent lack of qualifications. In my experience, these administrators are easier to win over than the many physicians who resent the power and authority of the physician-executive. Acknowledging their expertise and your own deficiencies and asking for their help are critical and are not, as might be initially feared, at all inconsistent with the authoritative style recommended earlier. Confidence and strength are required to know and own one's limitations. Since people expect physicians to be egotists, a bit of honest humility goes a long way, especially when the truth of such an attitude is so apparent. In order to succeed as a CEO of any organization, one must work effectively with senior managers. An additional benefit of working closely with one's senior staff is the likelihood that an open, trusting relationship with this group will become one of the few opportunities the physician-executive can count on for positive interpersonal experiences within the organization.

At the close of Part Three, Dr. Fernandez discusses three of the special challenges physician-executives face: the lack of immediate feedback on the results of decisions, the impossibility of pleasing all physicians at all times, and the uncertainty inherent in many management decisions. An additional concern that he describes may be easier to avoid: the belief that "I must accept ultimate blame for all the failures in the organization." Although CEO's must, of course, be willing to accept responsibility for all failures, they are hardly at fault, any more than they would be responsible for all successes. The recommendation to work closely with a highly effective senior-management team is the best antidote to feeling so overwhelmingly responsible.

We cannot avoid the other three problems, only understand them. Being a physician-CEO, particularly in an organization as fundamentally strong as the Nalle Clinic, is not so much like being a physician for a sick patient as it is like providing anticipatory guidance or health-maintenance advice to a patient experiencing normal growing pains. The rewards of preventive medicine are also in the distant future and require the physician's unwavering belief that the efforts are worthwhile in the absence of observable results. Dr. Fernandez's profound statement that "by the time I have made ten decisions, I have irritated everyone" shows that black humor, long an ally of physicians who need to learn to deal with death, is equally helpful to the physician-executive. This experience must be particularly difficult for someone like Dr. Fernandez, who believes that his "strongest skill was probably in being able to soothe troubled waters."

Finally, a CEO must deal with uncertainty. The reality of most senior-management decisions is that someone has already made the easy ones by the time an issue comes to your attention. You must use inadequate data for a much higher percentage of these decisions than in your experience as a physician. The ability to manage ambiguity and uncertainty is a critical quality for successful CEO's. However, in light of his statement that "we've got to keep telling our troops where we are taking them," the medical model may be hurting Dr. Fernandez. At times, if physicians fairly present alternatives and the risks and benefits of the approaches they choose, they may assure patients that a treatment will work out for the best even if they are less certain than that. This false certainty is seldom a useful approach for a CEO, particularly so in organizations driven by physicians who, as was noted earlier, are among the most difficult patients to manage.

Some of the openness and honesty with the physicians that Irv Rubin recommends in his first commentary on this section can be helpful. Paradoxically, when CEO's admit that they are uncertain about the best course to take, the effect can be to energize other staff—in this case, physicians in particular—to take more responsibility for decision-making, thereby decreasing their feelings of unhealthy dependency. This effect also precludes others from punishing the CEO for so-called failure (the only real failure is not learning from our experiences), since many people are involved.

We can hardly consider the experiences of the Nalle Clinic and Dr. Fernandez as failures. Their patients received good care. The organization grew and changed. Dr. Fernandez knows much more about management than he did ten years ago. And thanks to his generously describing these experiences, so do the rest of us. Stage-I physician-organizations all over the country have repeated the Clinic's story for the past decade and will continue to do so for another decade, as more and more of them evolve into successful Stage-II organizations in order to survive in an increasingly complex environment. The best of these will go on to excellence, to Stage III.

To help ourselves in this evolution, we must learn what we can from the teaching moments available to us, and this case gives us such an opportunity. A review of Dr. Fernandez's comments shows a recurrent theme. At various times he feels

> like a physician treating a Jehovah's Witness, knowing "that the patient is not able to accept advice, but we feel we've got to give the advice anyway";

> like Columbus: "most people actually hope we'll fall off the end of the world";

> and like a general "having to order some of his troops to storm a hill, absolutely knowing full well in advance that a lot of them are going to get shot and killed."[13]

Family therapists talk of "the identified patient," who commonly turns out to be the member of the family who is the most sensitive and intuitive and who acts out the family's unconscious wishes. Dr. Fernandez assumed this role for the Nalle Clinic. He describes himself as being a translator and a communicator. He sees the Board choosing him because of his lack of experience, because they could trust him not to upset the apple cart. His metaphors all deal with failure and loss and seem to represent what the Clinic needed of its leader during that period of its evolution.

A number of health-policy experts believe that group practices are the kind of medical organization in the best position to take advantage of the changes that are occurring in the business of providing and financing health care in the United States at this time. But to fulfill this role, these physician-led organizations will need to choose as their leaders those who they hope will succeed, not those whom they can count on to fulfill their unconscious need to resist change. Physician-managers who have gone through the kind of trial by fire that Dr. Fernandez has experienced and who have learned as much as he has will be ideal candidates for positions of leadership in organizations striving for excellence.

---

[13] The quotation is from a tape dictated after the announcement of the Clinic's merger with PhyCor. See p. 94 for the text.

COMMENTARY: FEELINGS IN TRANSITION

by Kevin Sullivan, M.D.
Vice President of Medical Affairs,
Port Huron Hospital

W hile reading a draft of this manuscript by Raymond Fernandez and Irv Rubin, I realized how little I had read about the feelings that accompany the transition to the role of physician-executive. Dr. Fernandez's open discussion (in Part Three) of his feelings as a physician-CEO encouraged me to express to him and to the reader some of the feelings that anyone is likely to encounter in making this journey into administration from the private practice of medicine.

Before deciding on a career as a physician-executive, you need to take a gut check of some important feelings. As a potential physician-executive, you must genuinely like and respect both physicians and administrators. Caring about the professional values and feelings of both will allow you to provide a buffer between them and to aid their communication with one another. If you are impatient or you hate meetings and paperwork, look for your career elsewhere. If you have a strong need to be in control, you feel uncomfortable working in teams, or you feel that consensus building is a waste of time, you will find most physician-executive positions frustrating. When physicians ask me whether they should consider careers as physician-executives, I take them through this gut check. The majority offer me condolences and say, "Thank God, I am a doctor."

But for some, like Dr. Fernandez, the challenge is right, and a whole new set of feelings surfaces. The importance and intensity of these feelings will vary by individual and by circumstances. A major feeling to deal with is that you have abandoned your patients, colleagues, and clinical practice. Dr. Fernandez felt this acutely: "Telling my patients and my peers that I had decided to leave them was emotionally trying, particularly with members of my call group." Both patients and colleagues want you and need you to care for them; colleagues need you to share call with them and be available for consultation. I did not feel right about becoming a full-time physician-executive until I had recruited my replacement to see my patients and to share call with my partner. At times when my patients say they wish I were still in practice, I wonder what the contract is that develops between physician and patient. "How can you give up all that residency training?" my father asked me. Not an easy question to answer. How do I explain walking away from skills I learned in four years of residency and strengthened in seventeen years of private practice?

Overcoming feelings of guilt and selfishness related to abandonment requires a strong commitment to the new vision and values of a Stage-III organization.

Another prevalent feeling is fear of the unknown. As Dr. Fernandez clearly articulated, the role of the physician-executive is to "have a clear vision of what is best for our organizations and where to lead them." Inevitably, you ask yourself, "Can I really make a difference in the organization by taking on this role? What if they don't like me and fire me? Can I afford to leave the financial security of private practice? Am I doing this for the right reasons, or am I just running away from the problems of private practice? Will I be happy and fulfilled in this new role?" To neutralize some of the fear of the unknown, I started as a part-time medical director. But ultimately, you have to take the plunge and live the answers. Dr. Fernandez correctly points out that you can't do justice to either job when you try to combine them.

You take the plunge. Then you face isolation. Some on the medical staff feel you have gone over to the dark side or, as Dr. Fernandez says, "feel you are a traitor." Some administrators wonder what value a physician adds to administration. In short, you face a credibility issue with both sides. Five years after taking the plunge, credibility still intact, I offer the following advice.

First, develop honest, open communication. Take to heart Dr. Fernandez's insight: "One of my most important duties is to translate and communicate others' ideas." A scheduled weekly meeting, not only with the administrative leaders but also with the medical leaders, is very helpful. We also developed a monthly meeting with senior management and the top medical leaders to improve communication and do some problem-solving. We send copies of important discussions with physicians to the chief of staff, the CEO, and the COO of our organization.

Second, identify the formal and informal physician-leaders, and get their buy-in for any major project that you want to implement. Doing this takes patience and the ability to educate, but the long-term result is well worth the effort. With stronger support from some of the influential physician-leaders of the Clinic, perhaps Dr. Fernandez could have avoided his feelings that "by the time I have made ten decisions, I have irritated everyone." At times, you still wonder what hat you wear. Can you really do justice to both medical-staff needs and administrative needs? At times, you feel ambivalence about whether you are being objective or leaning toward one side or the other.

Another feeling that is likely to surface is frustration that you lack both the information and management skills necessary to be a successful physician-executive. We spend years in medical education before becoming physicians, and we would be mistaken to think that we can get by with less than a major educational effort in the transition to management. As Dr. Fernandez points out, excellent educational opportunities exist. The American College of Physician Executives' Institute's courses and its series of Physicians-in-Management programs are helpful in developing operational managerial skills. The Estes Park seminars bring together physicians, board members, and administrators to hear and discuss the global issues that affect health care. Horty and Springer's seminars present the legal aspects of everything from medical-staff bylaws to joint ventures. These examples represent only a fraction of the educational opportunities available to physician-executives. The important thing to understand is that to avoid frustration and potential failure, you need an intense, ongoing educational effort.

Despite the finest educational experiences, most of the learning experience is on-the-job training and learning from your mistakes. This experiential growth in leadership skills and vision can help a physician-executive lead the organization to its next stage of development.

How do I feel about being a physician-executive? I love it. I love the challenges of helping physicians and administrators work together to develop the clinical and administrative systems that will reshape health care in our community. I feel renewed and energized. At times I miss the direct patient contact, but for me, the plunge has been worthwhile.

I have mixed feelings about Dr. Fernandez and his experience at the Nalle Clinic. I was uncomfortable with the adversarial relationships that developed at the Clinic between the physician-CEO and the organization. Does the physician-CEO have to feel, as Dr. Fernandez felt, like a general who must lose some of the troops to win the war?[14] I hope we can develop less war-like processes to change organizational cultures. I see on the horizon the principles of total quality management and trainings (such as Temenos's® *ABCs of Win-Win Relationships*), helping physician-CEO's and their organizations to deal with each other in a healthier manner.

On the other hand, I say to Dr. Fernandez, "Job well done! You facilitated the critical transition of the Nalle Clinic into a Stage-II organization. Your articulation of your role and feelings during this transition will be of great value to the physician-executives who follow in your footsteps."

---

[14] See p. 94 for quotation.

COMMENTARY:
THE LEGAL NUTS AND BOLTS OF TRANSITION

by Keith Korenchuk
Partner
Parker, Poe, Adams & Bernstein

While the Nalle Clinic had had a relationship with its law firm since at least 1950, the nature and level of services had been sporadic. In 1982 the Clinic, sensing a need for a more businesslike approach to its affairs, expressed a desire for a "more pro-active" approach from its lawyers. I joined the firm in the fall of that year, beginning my professional relationship with the Clinic and its new Medical Director, Ray Fernandez.

As the Clinic changed from a Stage-I to a Stage-II organization, I was a participant, not a neutral observer. Commenting on this transition, I benefit from hindsight and from my current role as a health-care attorney representing many medical groups.

Stage-I organizations, whether called by that name, or termed "medical condominiums" or "cottage industries," have a variety of common legal characteristics. First, these organizations typically employ their physicians through employment contracts that are written from the individual's perspective rather than the group's. In many ways these documents express the concept that the medical group is merely a collection of individuals whose rights are protected at the expense of the group's rights. These contracts result from physicians' desires to protect their compensation, benefits, and autonomy. The legal work is often prepared by an attorney who is a personal friend of individual physicians rather than by a law firm representing the group as a whole. Second, restrictive covenants, a mechanism whereby the group protects itself against potential competition created from within, are often nonexistent or not comprehensively drafted. Again, individual interests and autonomy are protected at the expense of the group. Third, group governance through its board of directors and a leadership team is often lacking or undeveloped. Many groups continue to operate as a pure democracy without defined leaders (ergo, anarchy), or, at the very least, a large and unworkable board which cannot make decisions on a timely basis. Thus, individual physicians in a Stage-I organization find it difficult to think of themselves as a group. The individual and his or her practice remain an autonomous entity.

Stage-II organizations typically exhibit an entirely different set of legal characteristics. First, employment agreements favor the group—for example, in decision-making. Second, restrictive covenants are accepted and recognized as a valuable tool for protecting the goodwill of the group. These covenants are comprehensively drafted to give the group every conceivable enforcement advantage. Finally, the board of directors develops into a small group with real decision-making authority. Since issues are fully developed with appropriate recommendations before they are presented to the board, meetings run efficiently.

In the early 1980's the Nalle Clinic exhibited classic Stage-I legal symptoms, yet it was already in transition. A major revision of the Clinic's employment relationships had strengthened the Clinic's group position. In addition, the Clinic recognized the need for more pro-active leadership, placing Dr. Fernandez in the role of Medical Director. These early initiatives, which may at the time have been viewed as final solutions, clearly represent just the initial attempts at change. These efforts were complicated by internal and external factors: costly computer conversions, declining morale, loss of revenue and staff, compensation and capitalization struggles, and competition from departed physicians and HMO's.

In 1984 and 1985 the Board and its Medical Director formulated plans during a retreat with Dr. Irv Rubin. The concept of an organization of excellence was adopted, and Dr. Fernandez was promoted to CEO. Had the Clinic not been confronted with these internal and external factors, the transition from a medical condominium to a Stage-II organization might have been accomplished according to plan. But because change cannot be statically implemented in a living, evolving organization, the Clinic detoured from its charted course.

Let's look at four issues facing the Nalle Clinic and its CEO. Each one illustrates a nuts-and-bolts difficulty of effecting change from a Stage-I to a Stage-II organization.

Issue One, Operation of the Board: In the early 1980's the Board had eleven members, all physicians. The large number created inefficiencies, and many physicians had difficulty giving up their individual autonomy in favor of group decision-making. The Board met in the evenings, routinely past 10 P.M., often until midnight. The meetings were sporadic. While members were concerned with results, discussions were unfocused. Preliminary discussions, development of alternatives, and consensus building were all done during the Board meeting, not before. With such a process, efficiency was low, frustration, high. This operation was classic Stage-I behavior.

At its retreat in 1984–85 the Board agreed to change its operating procedure from the medical-fraternity model. The size of the Board was decreased, thereby centralizing authority. Meetings were moved from the evening to the morning, when minds were fresh and when the press of a full day of medical practice would require efficient thinking and decision making. Finally, lay representatives were added to provide business expertise.

These changes looked good on paper, but were difficult to implement for several reasons. First, the pace of change accelerated, making it difficult, if not impossible, for the Board to complete its agenda in its allotted two hours per month. Second, individual physician Board members had difficulty separating their personal positions from that of the Clinic as a whole. Third, lay Board members did not integrate well with the physician majority. On one hand, physicians were convinced that the lay business people did not understand that medicine was a unique business in which patients must come first. On the other hand, the business people were as firmly convinced that physicians were incapable of making sound fiscal decisions, such as reducing compensation or cutting expenses to solve the Clinic's financial problems.

While much of the framework for transformation to a Stage-II board was in place in 1985, the PhyCor transaction itself provided the crisis from which the impetus to overcome inertia evolved. Lay Board members and physician members who did not embrace the group concept resigned, resulting in a strong core leadership that became convinced that the PhyCor partnership was in the best long-term interests of the Clinic. This core group, led by Dr. Fernandez, provided the necessary guidance and encouragement to its staff members, enabling the Clinic physicians to enthusiastically adopt the PhyCor alternative.

The new Stage-II Board is composed of equal members of PhyCor and the medical group. The Board continuously confronts new challenges. Leadership, organization, and decision-making remain critical for the Board, the Medical Director, and CEO. The painful experiences of moving from Stage I were not in vain, and the benefits of arriving at Stage II will not be lost.

Issue Two, Stock Ownership in the Clinic: For many years the physicians struggled with how the Clinic should be owned and who should vote for its Board. Historically, physicians used a percentage of their income to purchase stock each year. Stock ownership created two rights: 1) it allowed a shareholder to elect the Board of Directors; and 2) it conveyed ownership in the assets of the Nalle Clinic. However, the stock valuation method did not give the physicians the benefit of any appreciating equity in their business. Physicians viewed stock ownership as something that was required as "dues," so they gave little thought to the capital needs of the corporation. This method of operation was not unusual for smaller medical groups, which viewed themselves as collections of individuals rather than as a group.

In the 1984–85 period, a new strategy allowed the Clinic to evolve from a collection of individuals to an institution. This strategy required all physicians to own sixty shares of stock by purchasing three shares a year. Physicians who owned over sixty shares were invited to resell them to the Clinic. By requiring three shares to be purchased each year, rather than requiring a certain percentage of income to be contributed, the Clinic decided that a physician's income should not dictate his or her ultimate equity position in the company. Voting rights also changed in the direction of equality. Ultimately, everyone who had been at the Clinic for twenty years would have an equal voice in operations, regardless of specialty or income.

Again, theory was one thing and practice, another. First, some physicians refused to sell their shares, leaving several senior physicians with a large number of shares and a disproportionate control over who was elected to the Board. Second, the three-shares-per-year rule created a slow process by which physicians were deemed equals. Third, physicians grumbled about the cost to their take-home income. (There was the expense of hiring a full-time medical director/CEO. In addition, as salaries were paid according to a formula, some star performers saw their paychecks slashed.) Finally, the three shares purchased each year was not a significant amount that would improve the Clinic's ability to raise capital. Thus, the initial attempt at supporting the transition to Stage II through stock ownership fell short.

The turmoil of 1989–90 provided an opportunity to further reorient the Clinic philosophy. In order to foster group cohesiveness, share ownership and voting for the Board were separated from the control of Clinic assets. With respect to stock ownership, physicians who became senior staff physicians could immediately become shareholders on the same basis as any other Clinic shareholder. This reorganization recognized that physicians who were granted senior staff status should have an equal vote in the governance of the group, thus becoming group members as opposed to individual shareholders. The Clinic sold much of its non-real-estate assets to PhyCor, thereby eliminating the need for shareholders to own them. In addition, the real-estate assets were removed from the Clinic itself and placed in a limited partnership composed of its physicians. This plan encouraged physicians to remain loyal to the institution. Finally, Stage-II status could be achieved by securing access to capital through the new financial partner, PhyCor.

In summary, changes begun in 1984–85 resulted in a sweeping change of the Clinic's asset and ownership strategy. Ultimately the Clinic transformed from a fraternity into an institutional-based health-care organization.

Issue Three, Restrictive Covenants: In the medical-condominium model, the restrictive covenant is disfavored because it inhibits individual mobility by protecting group viability. In the early 1980's individual physicians at the Clinic were suspicious of restrictive covenants, viewing them as an intrusion on their ability to practice medicine. While the Clinic had instituted restrictive covenants in its contracts, they were prepared in such a way as to favor the individual at the expense of the group. In addition, the physician Board members retained their individual perspective in evaluating restrictive covenants. The value of restrictive covenants in protecting the goodwill of the group was often overlooked. Often the Board was reluctant to enforce a covenant, favoring a negotiated exit arrangement that inevitably resulted in the creation of a competitor who often had received his or her start by tapping into the goodwill of the Nalle Clinic. Costs mounted as physicians departed, taking patients with them. The associated costs in recruitment, lost revenue, and lost market share created serious financial consequences. In spite of mounting concern that physician departures impaired the group, little was done to strengthen enforcement policies. The Clinic also retained its long-standing policy that physicians with ten years of service were no longer subject to the restrictive covenants.

The catalyst for Stage-II change in restrictive covenants was PhyCor. PhyCor required that all Clinic physicians, new and established, execute significantly more comprehensive agreements. Business considerations dictated that stronger enforcement practices now be implemented. The covenants limited individual freedom to practice in exchange for a benefit in strengthening the organization. The Board and its Medical Director recognized that restrictive covenants had a significant role in making divorce a less easily taken route in resolving disputes. It is clear that, with PhyCor's assistance and in light of the experience with no-fault divorce in the late 1980's, the medical group achieved a Stage-II view of the role of a restrictive covenant.

Issue Four, Role of the CEO: As discussed previously, the Nalle Clinic had difficulty defining the role for its physician-CEO. Like many patients, the Clinic found it difficult to define for its caregiver where it hurt, so the CEO was constantly evaluating his patient. He wore different hats with different groups. To the Stage-I Board, the CEO often played an implementing role, waiting for instructions before acting. This role slowly evolved to a leadership position. To individual physicians the CEO was a communicator and a lightning rod for frustrations. To consultants the CEO was the healer and advocate, conscious of what was needed by his patient, the Clinic.

In treating his patient in 1989, Dr. Fernandez recognized that both internal and external factors were impeding the transition to Stage II (though he might not have called it that), and he became convinced that the most viable strategy was to implement the PhyCor relationship and to make sure it succeeded, even though that success meant a change in his own role as CEO. However, in my view, this process was not at all like Dr. Fernandez's statement that "the patient was referred to a specialist." Clearly, without his own leadership in the evaluation, analysis, and implementation of the PhyCor agreement, the Clinic's evolution to Stage II would not have occurred so quickly. One who was so in touch with his patient and who was continuously involved in hands-on care was the real "specialist." The CEO was able to conclude that PhyCor represented a vehicle for achieving organizational change. While the Medical Director-CEO became Medical Director in the process, the strategy helped his patient through a temporary illness, and led to a group-practice transformation.

Conclusion: To survive and prosper, medical groups must confront the transition from a bunch of individuals to a cohesive group. This change is not a total transformation; it is a shift in the balance of power. Each group must require its individuals to trust the group more, to surrender their individual rights for the common good, and to subscribe to the group mission. Different individual interests will always create tension in organizations, so effecting change inevitably creates adversarial relationships. Those who propose change must be prepared for resistance from those who do not want to change. The challenge for medical-practice leaders, one successfully faced by Dr. Fernandez, is to channel that change, to evaluate the patient, and to implement strategies that work. Groups which make this transition have bright futures. As this case study of the Nalle Clinic has shown, successful implementation may require a variety of strategies, some of which can only be discerned after the process is well under way. The ability to understand and implement the necessary legal transformation to Stage-II behavior is vital to a leader's fulfillment of his duty to his patient.

COMMENTARY:
THE PATIENT SPEAKS

by John L. Benedum, M.D.
President of the Nalle Clinic Board of Directors

Editor's Note: While we have entitled this brief commentary "The Patient Speaks," it would be inappropriate and unfair to presume that any single individual can speak for the entire Nalle Clinic. Many years together in the trenches have brought Dr. Fernandez and Dr. Benedum to a treasured level of mutual trust and respect. While some of Dr. Benedum's observations from the patient's perspective might be seen by others as critical, they are offered and received as gifts of genuine caring. Such is the power of win-win relationships among valued friends and colleagues, among providers and patients. Without honest, direct, heart-to-heart feedback, there can be little learning, growth, development, and healing.

This patient-organization is well known to me. I joined the Nalle Clinic in 1979 as one of the first two general internists added to the group. Two years later I was elected to the governing Board of Directors. I had a keen interest in guiding the direction of the Clinic and represented a primary-care constituency. Through the years described in the Case Report, I was an active observer and participant in those changes. I would like to share my perspective on the Clinic and the career of my colleague, friend, and attending physician, Ray Fernandez.

The Nalle Clinic was Charlotte's only significant health-care group, outside of the hospitals, in the early 1980's. We invested a great deal of energy, time, and money to restructuring our decision-making processes and administrative roles. I recall considerable skepticism and resistance from many members of the group. Organizational psychology and management terminology were foreign to most of us on the Board of Directors. Admittedly, we were much less comfortable in these roles compared to our more traditional physician roles. For example, it was a monumental effort to achieve consensus on the mission of this developing organization!

We spent so much time reorganizing and positioning ourselves for a future that we thought was going to be more competitive and more demanding that we failed to nurture and accommodate some factions within the group. The Clinic's leadership decided that the interests of the whole organization came first. Unable to see the future benefits of this investment in a growing organization, some physicians and departments left the Clinic. Their retreat to simpler, single-specialty practices compounded our financial stresses and undermined our spirit.

The decision to hire a part-time Medical Director from within the ranks of the Clinic, someone we all knew and trusted, speaks to the caution with which we were testing these new waters. The Board had a list of chores that they thought would be best done by a physician: being a liaison between physicians and administration, recruiting new staff and negotiating their contracts, and co-ordinating physician committees. The role of the Medical Director and then the Medical Director/CEO developed around Dr. Fernandez, his personality and skills.

In the care of a patient with an identified illness, there are standards of care and an accepted treatment plan. In a changing medical environment, the course that our medical group should take was not clear to any of us. We assigned a formidable task to our physician colleague. He agreed to trade quick feedback and appreciation from his patient interactions (his patients miss him yet today), for an often hostile environment where gratification is, at best, delayed or often non-existent.

As we all became more comfortable thinking of the organization as having a life of its own, it became easier to delineate responsibilities and authority to administrative team members. By virtue of his devotion, energies, and communication skills, Dr. Fernandez became the natural leader in this transition period. He had his critics, for sure, but with patience and persuasion he guided the organization toward a more efficient structure. Physicians and the Board gradually seemed more willing to relinquish some of their individual control in the best interests of the group. There was never a ground swell of unanimous support. Some physicians stated emphatically that this was not the Clinic that they had joined and that they could no longer live with this new direction and its influences on their autonomy and style of practice.

Slowly and cautiously, changes occurred. We were still unwilling to make dramatic changes in personnel and business practices. Dr. Fernandez, the officers and the Board of Directors shared responsibility for decisions leading to the increasing financial problems. In retrospect, however, I wonder if our organization would have survived the challenges of 1988–89 had we not restructured. Even at that point, many of us were still clinging to the idea that the situation would improve and things would work out. They always had in the past! To chart our course and move confidently into an uncertain future, we kept searching for more data, better data, more inspirational leadership, and more expert analysis. If we could only find that visionary who possessed all the other executive qualities, surely we could weather this storm. We began to search for a more experienced, hard-nosed, detail-oriented administrator to complement Dr. Fernandez's visionary, soft style. My interpretation of the feelings of several Board members and physicians was that, although Dr. Fernandez was appreciated for his ability to listen and to resolve conflicts, he was not capable of critically analyzing the financial data. I think that he did not get creative solutions or adequate analysis from his administrative staff and was unwilling to change that management team significantly. As our back-office operations and systems were obviously unsuccessful, we had an even greater need of a strong-handed turnaround expert.

It seems clear to me now that this problem developed over several years. We hire, train, and reward administrators to be subservient to the physician-run corporation. Then we criticize them when they speak their own mind. At the same time, we physicians are going along with our day-to-day routine and busy practices, assuming that someone is minding the store . . . until something upsets our personal worlds. I don't think the physician Board members or the administration stayed abreast of our financial situation. When the crisis flared up, Dr. Fernandez took most of the heat. Perhaps this was appropriate. To his credit, he remained poised and professional. He did not panic when his patient was hemorrhaging.

The organization was slowly maturing, but we felt a sense of urgency in the summer of 1989. Rather than dismiss Dr. Fernandez, as some urged, we agreed to search for a savior. The death of the Nalle Clinic as a multispecialty group was considered only as a last resort. We looked locally and we hired a search firm. Those unsuccessful efforts and our lack of confidence in our own abilities to turn the business around fueled our search for a corporate partner. I suggested looking outside the medical field because I thought that such business expertise did not exist in traditional clinic settings.

To Dr. Fernandez's credit, he initiated and participated in a search for a partner who could provide the necessary capital and business expertise. With PhyCor came a renewed hope, energy, and a recovery of our confidence in the Clinic: with the new personnel and capital, we would be able to achieve our goals.

COMMENTARY:
A MARKETING CONSULTANT'S PERSPECTIVE

by Bruce Fritch
President of Fritch Consulting
Charlotte, North Carolina

T he physicians at the Nalle Clinic were bright, earnest physicians, successful and proud in their individual practices. Why did they experience so much difficulty and turmoil when facing the challenges of a mutual purpose? What can we learn from this extraordinary case study that can help us avoid its pitfalls? Is it reasonable to work toward the quality patient-care standards of Japan's St. Marguerite Hospital and still hope to achieve attractive profitability goals?

Preview

In this commentary I will relate the case of the Nalle Clinic and perhaps Every Clinic to factors which are contributing to the persistence of dysfunctional Stage-I phenomena. I will point to the importance of power in relationships and to our responsibility for shaping the quality of relationships. For it isn't enough to understand the characteristics of Stages I, II, and III. We must learn to build transition bridges from one to the other.

It is possible to build a profitable, quality-oriented group practice with a strategy that encompasses profit as well as standards of medical competence and patient care. Shaping such an organization begins with the personal influence of the chief executive officer *and* the board of directors, department managers, and professional and lay staffs. The whole organization must have several ingredients: a mutual purpose, an acceptance of their intense interdependence, and the will and the skill to resolve the inevitable conflicts and frustrations that arise. Most important, it must take action. Initially what we as individual practitioners can do is increase our interpersonal skills and awareness, our effectiveness as *leaders*. We must strengthen the quality of our relationships within the marketplace (with patients and referring physicians), and within our professional organizations today.

The Phenomena of Power and Influence

Let's begin by looking at John French and Bertram Raven's[15] widely regarded

---

[15] "The Bases of Social Power," in *Group Dynamics: Research and Theory,* 3rd ed., ed. by Dorwin Cartwright and Alvin Zander, (New York: Harper & Row, 1968), pp. 262–268. Originally published in *Studies in Social Power,* D. Cartwright, ed. (Ann Arbor, Mich.: Institute for Social Research, 1959).

model describing five common bases of power: reward, coercive, referent, legitimate, and expert. Of these, legitimate and expert are most relevant here.

Legitimate power is based on people's belief that *agents* of authority (for example, government or a CEO), have a legitimate right to prescribe behavior for them. Legitimate power stems from values we internalized growing up. It manifests in our belief that someone or some group has the "legitimate right to influence" a person, and that that person has an *"obligation* [italics added] to accept this influence."[16] While factors such as age, intelligence, and physical characteristics may influence legitimate power, it is often bestowed on someone by an empowering licensing agency. For example, the AMA, state medical boards, and medical schools are legitimizing agencies of authority. With legitimate power, the extent of the authority is generally specified when the power is designated (for example, the conferring of Board Certification). If actions extend outside this authority, explicit resistance and a decrease in power is likely (as we have seen when schools boards attempted to censor classroom books).

Expert power originates from having superior knowledge or ability in specific areas. The strength of expert power "varies with the extent of knowledge or perception" of knowledge which a person attributes to the agent of authority.[17] Several requirements are at work:

1. Others must have confidence that the expert has knowledge.
2. Expert power is restricted to a given field of expertise. Although there may be a halo effect (evidenced by the number of star athletes who promote breakfast cereals or underwear), most expert power is limited. When others conclude that the expert is out of line, "an undermining of confidence seems to take place."[18]
3. Others must perceive that the expert is trustworthy—credible and reliable. Trust builds over time by doing the little things right all of the time. If the little things are neglected, a negative halo effect can occur. For example, airlines that don't clean coffee stains from tray tables can contribute to a moment of passenger anxiety about the quality of engine maintenance. Similarly, physicians who can't keep their appointment-time promises contribute to the discontent (dis-ease) of their patients.

What's Happening to the Regard for Authority?

Authority is most simply defined as "the ability to get a desired response to one's wishes." No desired response, no authority. Hence, authority is power of the most

---

[16] *Ibid.* p. 265.

[17] *Ibid.* p. 267.

[18] *Ibid.* p. 268.

practical sort, influencing demand for services and professional relationships alike. In the past we *automatically* depended on our experts. But the fundamental nature of how people relate to authority has changed.

Since World War II, Americans have become skeptical, even cynical, of authority. Many events have contributed to the change, including Watergate, computerized trading scandals, hazardous waste accumulation, and exposure of inept public officials and immoral evangelists. The change is reflected in the civil rights movement, contraception, feminism, government watch-dog committees, and voter apathy.

Not until the Vietnam War did attitudes begin to shift on a large scale, considerably fostered and conveyed by the news media. Americans questioned the morality of being in Vietnam; the competence of military and political leaders to wage an effective war; and the ethics and honesty of the media, the military, and the government. The effect was protests and marches, rocks and tear gas. There was a tremendous polarization in regard for traditional authority.

Other factors amplified the change in public regard for authority: the news media (performing as news makers, rather than news reporters); microcomputers and other high-tech, intelligence-enhancing tools (placing the power of information and technology into the hands of the many); and terrorism and the assassinations of President Kennedy, Bobby Kennedy, and Martin Luther King, Jr. (weakening the public's faith in authorities' ability to protect and defend).

Skepticism grew in the 1980's. Changes in public regard for authority exploded world wide. From brave efforts by Polish shipyard workers to the bitter response to political and social incompetence in Rumania, to Soviet *Glasnost*, to resisting apartheid in South Africa, people are insisting on new relationships with authorities and are setting aside those which are fundamentally unequal or disrespectful.

I think the changes in the public's regard for authority, with the commensurate demand for relationships of greater quality, is the most significant factor influencing the effectiveness of professional organizations today. I have seen its growth in the health-care marketplace since the mid-1980's. And it is evolving in other professional services markets, such as accounting and management consulting. Now the impact on health-care organizations is particularly dramatic.

A Perspective for Viewing: A New Consumerism

Over the past decade a new consumerism has been evolving, aimed at relationships in the professions. It is based on skepticism about professionals and an unwillingness to tolerate behavior, intentional or not, that diminishes the consumer's self-esteem. New-consumer patients want to be treated as persons, not just as a body of symptoms. The appearance of a white coat does not convey carte-blanche authority. They challenge the medical experts' diagnoses, fees, and range of authority.

The sports and fitness movement has been especially pivotal in shaping a new view of physicians. Millions of tennis, running, and exercise buffs began reading about exercise, nutrition, and fitness. Visiting their physicians, they seized the opportunity to verify the tips they had acquired. Too many discovered that their physicians' knowledge of wellness was inadequate. This perception was amplified if these doctors smoked or were overweight, and did not practice what they preached. As a result, skepticism and doubt encroached on these patients' traditionally compliant attitudes.

The self-help movement further eroded the dependence on physician authority. As people learned to take greater responsibility for their own well-being, they came face to face with the humanness of their healers. Patients, such as Norman Cousins, who wrote *Anatomy of an Illness*, discovered that they could contribute to their own health as much as, or more than, physicians.

The new consumerism entails a change in the relationship with authorities, both legitimate and expert. The confidence and trustworthiness necessary for expert power must be regained through a team relationship. Today, if patients don't experience the relationship or medical quality they expect, they are likely to seek help elsewhere.

Power Dynamics in Physician-Patient Relationships

With the expert power of miracle drugs and space-age technology at their disposal, doctors have been accused of having a superior attitude, a priestly mien. Sometimes this is characterized by the lack of information that physicians communicate to patients. Lack of communication, whether from physician to patient or to referring physician, can be interpreted as deceitful. Patients conclude that too often there is a lack of respect: physician as priest, patient as child.

Curiously, physicians tell me they rarely see it this way. "Respect patients? Of course I respect my patients!"—as though the suggestion were absurd. Juggling new technologies, competitive pressures, and third-party payment guidelines, physicians are called on to accept one more challenge, that of assertive, unsolicitous patients.

Patients, especially those over 55 years old, have done their part to maintain the priestly mien by behaving subserviently with their doctors. They didn't question why their doctors did not meet their needs for information and availability.

Recently a 71-year-old woman, complaining of sore legs and excessive fatigue, visited her doctor. Sitting in an examination room, her resting pulse was 143. The physician ordered her into the hospital where she was extensively tested for three days and nights, treated according to findings, and released on drug therapy. Her children—ages 32, 43, and 45, who lived out of state—persistently inquired about her condition. The woman, all the while pleased with her physician, could never offer an informed response. She had not been told, and she was reluctant to inquire for information that the doctor had not volunteered. If the doctor had wanted her to know, she thought, he would have told her.

Who was right? Her adult children were infuriated, vowing never to let a physician get away with such disrespect and so-called treatment. To them, the quality of the physician's relationship with their mother was inappropriate. Some readers will argue that if the physician had offered treatment and met the patient's expectations, then the physician acted appropriately. Another issue, however, is how future patients (e.g., the three adult children), will respond to the same treatment. *What is the right thing for the physician to do?* The quality of the relationship is of growing importance in the marketplace.

However, we must not lose sight of the point that market share is a result. The purpose of improving the relationship is improving the quality of care. In spirit, the new consumerism is reminding the profession of the Hippocratic Oath: "In every house where I come, I will enter only for the good of my patients."

It is a massive overstatement that physicians have a genetic, personality-driven, or med-school-instilled propensity to be uninformative, unavailable, and unresponsive. Regardless of the reason, many of us recognize that another dynamic is operating. The malpractice mania and doctor bashing we are seeing is being caused, psychologically, by a sense that a fiduciary trust has been broken. Isn't it curious that my old family doctor knew less and had less technology than today's experts, yet we trusted him implicitly? Why would it never have occurred to my parents to sue him even if he made a lethal mistake? This is the kind of issue that I believe needs more careful attention.

M.D.'s are not, in my view, sole causal agents. Like all of us, they are caught in a living dynamic transformation. The change in how people relate to authority is purging the priestly mien from physicians' choices of acceptable attitudes. This change makes it impossible, as well as undesirable, for physicians to focus only on the quality of their technology and their competence at their craft, devoting little effort or awareness to the quality of their professional relationships. Because of the significance of their roles in society, we look to physicians to embrace a leadership challenge: to first heal themselves.

Recommendations for Symptoms of Ineffective Patient Relationships

Trust is essential in a physician-patient relationship. Because of circumstances of illness, one party is more helpless than the other party. The unique challenge to many professional relationships is that the situation puts one party in a one-down position. This challenges the helper to (a) accept the other's helplessness as being real while (b) still treating the other as a full person. And it is the helper's professional responsibility (fiduciary trust) to take the initiative and to be helpful. Here, help is evaluated from the perspective of the party being helped. The challenge is great. Who among us finds it easy to be informative, available, and responsive to a person who, in his or her position as patient, represents a potential malpractice threat or production inefficiency?

To heal the relationships, physicians must consciously demonstrate their care and compassion for each patient. New-consumer patients want their physicians to be teammates, partners in health. As we will see in the next sections, collaborative team-work can become the theme of the authority relationships in the 1990's.

Power Dynamics in Physician-Group Relationships

Physicians' relationships with legitimate power (represented to the physicians within their organizations by the CEO, the board, and the administration) have been changing, too. Reflecting a new consumerism of their own, physicians also express, and react to, legitimate and expert power in very significant ways. In particular, physicians are less willing to let others govern the organization without receiving information and assurances from those in charge. Changes in the relationship that physicians experience within their own organizational environment parallel the changes discussed here in physician-patient relationships. The point is, the shift in regard for authority applies equally.

Summary of the Nalle Clinic Situation in the 1980's

Bursting with Stage-I energy, the Nalle Clinic was the quintessential fraternity model. Yet fraternal it was not. Despite the efficient and professional conduct of physicians in their individual practices, the collective team of physicians did not work together effectively. Forces of the self-centered traits typical of a Stage-I organization were stronger than the attractions of mutual purpose and high-quality teamwork. Driving these Stage-I behaviors was the physician at odds with the Clinic's legitimate authority: the Board and especially the CEO (legitimate power personified).

Lacking confidence in management's expertise, the physician group frustrated *itself* with the lack of decision-making progress. Administrative and Board-level decisions were delayed until the assembled all-physician staff (nearly 80!) could debate and determine the course of action (about one meeting per month). Predictably, personal agendas intruded on organizational purposes; divisiveness stamped out interdependence. Executive appropriateness was based more on con-formity with the wishes of the all-physician staff than on accepted standards of man-agement. In particular, appropriateness was rarely based on the decision of those nominally responsible for decision making (i.e., the CEO, Board, and administra-tors). Second-guessing by the all-physician staff resulted in paralysis in daily admin-istrative and operational decision making. This paralysis spread to the Board of

Directors, inhibiting their ability to deal with policy issues.

A lack of interpersonal skills and a lack of organizational effectiveness in such Stage-I groups is understandable. What medical school emphasizes relationship philosophy and skills? Physicians' training focuses on knowledge, tools, and craft—on the hard sciences of medicine and not on the softer, interpersonal arts of healing. What is the root cause of physician behavior that others experience as abusive to self-esteem? Recent research has put it at the hands and feet of physicians' teachers.[19] In other words, physicians are just practicing what they learned. It is the managers and executives in non-medical business organizations who receive extensive human-development training.[20] It is only the most enlightened of physicians and physician-executives who create time in their busy schedules for interpersonal skill-building training. For health-care organizations in the 1990's this, *too*, must change.

Recommendations for Treating Symptoms of Organizational Ineffectiveness

Step 1. Administrators and physicians must learn to appreciate and respect their differences. One group has a heart-felt understanding of the operation of a business; and the other, of the business of operations. They need each other to achieve their heart-felt mutual purpose: providing quality care.

Step 2. Physicians, as leaders, must develop their interpersonal skills. On-the-job learning will be necessary. When physicians and administrators attend seminars together on management and systems of monitoring quality care, they report, "We now understand each other better."

Step 3. Physicians must demonstrate greater respect and a willingness to learn from others. The physician staff at Every Clinic must attempt to understand and implement the recommendations of their committees who have done careful research. In the same spirit, administrators must respect physicians' ability and desire to learn about management and organizational leadership.

These philosophies, skills, and perspectives all transfer to relationships with patients and referring physicians. As a direct consequence, they will affect the bottom line. Yes, we can have the quality patient care of Japan's St. Marguerite along with business prosperity. The physician group that is willing to strive toward a mutual purpose, work as a team, and abide by high-performance team agreements can bridge to Stage II.

---

[19] Henry K. Silver, M.D. and Anita Duhl Glickens, M.S.W., "Medical Student Abuse: Incidence, Severity, and Significance," *JAMA*, 263, no. 4, (January 26, 1990), pp. 527–537.

[20] For a discussion of the link between quality improvement and behavior toward customers, see Irwin Rubin and Robert Inguagiato, "Behavioral Quality Assurance: A Transforming Experience," *Physician Executive*, 16, no. 5 (Sept.–Oct. 1990), pp. 30–33.

The Action Steps to Recovery

Knowledge about what needs improvement is not a mystery to any doctor, lawyer, or chief executive. The steps to recovery are specific:

1. Admit that what we have is not good enough, not working well enough, yet.
2. Stop doing what we've done in the past that we know is not helping.
3. Decide together with colleagues what has to be done. We will have to learn how to do some of the things we know we need to do, and we will need to practice daily, preferably together.

As long as we allow ourselves to be distracted from our mutual primary purpose, our dependent patients have no choice but to continue to struggle to get our attention with any means at their disposal. Until we learn to work together as a quality team, we have no right to expect any more from our patients.

Our regard for authority has been changing. We can expect it to evolve into this decade and beyond. Responding sufficiently in the areas of human relations and team building will be physicians'—professionals'—performance challenge of the 1990's.

COMMENTARY:
TURBULENT PASSAGES OF CHANGE AND THE DYNAMICS OF POWER

by Irwin Rubin, Ph.D.

Who is the speaker here, and who is being accused?

"You don't fully explain the reasons for your decisions."
"You use jargon instead of simple language I can understand."
"You're difficult to reach by phone."
"You're hard to get an appointment with."
"You treat me like a little child, not an adult."
"You're more concerned about money than about quality care."

The most common response is "patients are accusing their physician providers." Surprise! There is another correct answer: "physicians are accusing their managerial providers." The motivation behind both sets of accusations is improvement in the quality of care. Yet allies are acting like enemies.

Power, and its redistribution and rebalancing, create strong emotional reactions. Many years ago I was working with a health-care organization that used an interdisciplinary team approach. Team-leader physicians resisted our team-building project because they feared that their power was about to be usurped. As one physician put it, "I don't have time or need for this touchy-feely stuff!" At the end of the project, he said with relief, "I still make 75% of the decisions on this team . . . but now I do it after consulting with my teammates!"

Reducing physicians' power—that is, reducing their responsibility for medical decisions—is not the objective. Expanding their power base, increasing their total sphere of influence, is one challenge. The second is to reframe our negative reaction to the word *power*. As we have seen in Bruce Fritch's commentary, deep forces in society have changed patients' relationship with expert power. No longer is the patient willing to passively swallow all the pills the physician prescribes. Psychologically, the current malpractice mania can be seen as the necessary, although painful and dysfunctional, counterdependent phase preceding a more adult-to-adult relationship.

Physicians are the common denominator in both answers to the flying accusations beginning this commentary. In one case, physicians are on the pointy end of the arrow; in the other, they are on the feather end. Adding TLC, the healing power of their whole persons, along with sophisticated intellects and technology will have two effects for physicians: (1) increasing the quality of care, and (2) developing both empathy and a win-win approach toward their managerial leadership. The healthier the organization, the greater the quality of care that patients receive. In other words, the change in the relationship we see as being necessary between M.D.'s and their patients will mirror the changes we see needing to occur in the relationship between physicians and administrators. This is one of the leadership challenges in health care, and physicians are the key.

Physicians as individuals, as dependent members of health-care organizations, express their changing regard for the authority of their providers in governance issues. The case of the Nalle Clinic demonstrates a power struggle taking place in many Stage-I fraternity organizations: physicians are less willing to let others govern the organization (make priestly pronouncements), without being informed. Their Stage-I level of maturity results in ambivalence, as Dr. Fernandez has noted:

> Although all physicians demanded "better management," their disdain for bureaucracy and administration intensified. Physicians did not volunteer to serve on the Board of Directors. Rather, like Monday morning quarterbacks, many knew exactly what plays should have been called. Few seemed willing to leave their seats on the 50-yard line and join the battle on the astroturf.[21]

We are not saying that teamwork has been totally absent from the relationship between physicians and their patients or between physicians and their managerial providers. Different kinds of teams are needed at various stages of development.[22] Power varies accordingly.

The balance of power shifts dramatically as organizations move from the Stage-I baseball team to the Stage-II football team to the Stage-III basketball team. Consider planning meetings. Meetings are a key forum for power plays; they're an arena where influence takes place. Specific rules prescribe how many people are allowed to meet on the pitcher's mound and how often. (Never 80 once a month!) A representative from the dugout, the head office, is only allowed one visit to these meetings before the pitcher's head must roll. When the team's on the field, other important communications (attempts at influence) must be yelled across the field or transmitted via coded body English.

By contrast, typically, no formal move is planned on a football team without a

---

[21] See p. 2.

[22] See pp. 42–3 for a discussion of the support that team members require to make the behavioral changes during major transitions, to learn how to play different games.

huddle of all the relevant team members. Shuttle diplomacy may operate as the coach sends in plays, but the entire team hears the word at the same time and has a chance to respond. ("I think I can beat him long with a 32X left!") The most respected and experienced quarterbacks are granted the legitimate power to use their expertise unilaterally (not autocratically), call an audible and change the play on the line of scrimmage.

As we have noted, basketball only works like magic when the meeting of the minds takes place "intuitively" or can be directed by one player while the game is being played. A basketball team, like a Stage-III organization, is less dependent on the power of supervision and more dependent on the power of Super Vision.

It is not enough to simply understand the characteristics of various stages of development as static steady states. We must also learn how to survive and grow together during the inevitably unsteady transitions between stages. Regardless of the context (parent and child, physician and patient, professional and employing organization), growing up is always associated with a shift in the balance of power. Learning to manage these dynamics begins with accepting some simple, though painful, truths about power and the process of change.

A counterbalancing of forces characterizes an organization in the steady state of existence, regardless of its particular stage of development. The forces pushing for change are met by virtually equal and opposite forces of resistance, which create an equilibrium. For example, younger employees interested in growth will support new capital expansion proposals ("Our future lies in growth"), while old-timers will resist ("I'm getting ready to retire. Don't burden me with any more debt load").

This process dynamic can be subtle. In deciding to elect a physician to a management position as medical director and asking him "to devote 50% of his time to administrative matters at a salary of 50% of the average physician's income," the Nalle Clinic added to the forces of change. The idea, as Dr. Fernandez noted, "was to financially motivate the medical director to improve the physicians' incomes." On the other hand, the Board created an equal and opposing force of resistance because it "did not spell out the position's power and authority [did not give Dr. Fernandez legitimate power], except to point out that the medical director would attend Board meetings in an advisory capacity but *would not vote*" [emphasis added]. The same passive-resistant dynamic operated when Dr. Fernandez was made full-time CEO, a potentially powerful position for change. He did not ask for a formal set of performance expectations, and the Board did not offer one. Neither he nor the Board would be able to know if he was making it or not.

So the stage was set for ambiguity and its by-product, fear. Imagine how the crews of the Niña, the Pinta, and the Santa Maria felt as they sailed through uncharted seas. Their CEO promised a brave new world, but the sailors believed they were doomed to fall off a flat earth!

Successful change rests upon reducing fear and resistance. Reducing, not eliminating. Change for change's sake can be as irresponsible as resistance for resistance's sake. I believe that change strategies that focus exclusively on the power of
increasing pressure will have high human costs. Logical explanations and data-
driven analyses to justify needed changes are necessary but insufficient. Emotional
support, TLC, is necessary to reduce this fear. For example, the fact that my physician had performed a particular surgical procedure successfully a thousand times
made my head happy, but did little to soothe my gut. I had the fleeting thought
that he was probably due for a failure! The fact that the professionally trained physician-managers and administrators have performed particular organizational procedures successfully in the past does little to reduce physicians' fears about who's
running the store.

More than they can admit, physicians today are gripped by fear and anxiety.
They are dependent on the system of an organization, a collective, to provide the
context, resources, and protection to allow them to do the job they trained for: caring for individual patients. They spend countless hours worrying about their
salaries, just as patients and insurance companies complain about rising costs. They
grumble about decisions made for them by others on high, just as patients resent
long waiting times and prescriptions written without sufficient explanation. In part
because they have not dealt with their own fears and anxieties, "many physicians
are unaware that patients experience 'massive amounts of anxiety' during sickness
and treatment."[23] This lack of awareness results in behaviors that patients think are
insensitive. For example, probing the body with a cold instrument without explain-
ing why, in terms they understand, can lead patients to conclude that their physician doesn't care. (Forcing budgets down physicians' throats causes gagging, too!)
Less physically intrusive, but no less insensitive, is the feeling many patients get
that "their time is worth nothing." They wait long periods for short visits that result
in huge bills.

Respect for clients can come from surprising sources. For example, a tire deal-
ership in Hawaii provides quality care to its customers. If customers are forced to
wait twenty minutes longer than the scheduled appointment time, they receive a
cash discount.

I recently visited my doctor for a follow-up appointment. I was asked the same
history questions ("Any history of heart trouble in your family? . . ."), that I had
answered three times the previous month. It was only when I objected that this waste
of my time stopped . . . but not before my trust eroded another tick.

A violated trust triggers a counterdependent reaction. In the medical profession

---

[23] Irwin Press, "The Predisposition to File Claims: The Patient's Perspective," *Law, Medicine & Health Care*,
April, 1984, p. 54.

this takes the form of malpractice mania. As medical researchers have documented,[24] factors often labeled as "the soft psychological stuff"—awareness, trust, and sensitivity—can directly impact the healing process.

Many years ago I observed physicians prescribing medication to Hispanic people living in the squalor of New York's South Bronx. These young, white, upper-class doctors said, "Take three times daily with regular meals." The look on these patients' faces seemed to say, "Yeah, as if I could afford to eat three times a day! Who are these guys in white coats? What do they know?" I saw several people drop their pills into the trash on their way out. To these patients, the doctors had no expert power. Medical research shows that 50-60% noncompliance is not uncommon.[25]

Comparable figures are not available vis-á-vis physicians-as-patients in response to managerial directives. As Dr. Fernandez noted in his Medical Record, however, "Members of the Clinic frequently appealed the decisions made by the Board and committees. Lengthy delays in making and implementing decisions became common. The Clinic never did implement certain decisions. Over a five-year period, two separate committees studied cost accounting, but the Clinic's members would not accept any of their proposals."[26]

High tech, be it sophisticated management information systems or M.R.I.'s (Magnetic Resonance Imaging), does little to reduce people's gut fear of change. Such high tech can actually increase fear. Regardless of how carefully experts explain their M.R.I., only the expert really knows how—or if—it works. What can reduce resistance and fear to manageable proportions? TLC. High touch. Higher touch means changing the nature and the quality of the *relationship* between physician and patients and between physicians and administrators. Dr. Fernandez anticipated this when he noted, "One of my most important duties is to translate and communicate others' ideas," to keep people in touch. He quickly added, "However, listeners tend to mistrust a translator they must depend on."[27]

Just as a lay person can not expect to become a medical expert by reading *Reader's Digest*, physicians can ill afford to shortchange the business of management by acting as if it were a profession that any bright, educated, earnest individual could learn overnight. Board meetings can no more be crammed into overscheduled patient hours than can complicated surgical procedures.

As educated consumers, we can ask good questions of our providers. *If* they take place in the context of a relationship based on mutual respect and trust, as opposed to attack and defensiveness, these questions can guide the efforts of our providers. Similarly, educated physicians can be supporters of their managerial providers if the

---

[24] *Ibid.*, pp. 53–62.

[25] *Ibid.*, p. 54.

[26] See p. 3.

[27] See p. 48.

same relationship of mutual respect and trust can be built.

Over a period of several years, a forward-thinking physician-CEO invited several hundred of his key physicians to attend a one-week, in-house seminar on management. Lay administrators were invited, too. It was a huge time investment. (You readers can tally the lost billable hours.) A personal invitation from the CEO was not easy to refuse, so many attended . . . with mixed feelings. Virtually everyone finished the seminar with a deeper appreciation for, and understanding of, the managerial role in the provision of quality care.

Instead of M.D.'s approaching their organization's managers like frightened, angry children fighting with their parents, they need to be helped to join with their colleagues in the creation of a team relationship. Physician-CEO's who can facilitate this shifting of collective power, this rebalancing, will be influencing the quality of the relationship between physicians (professionals) and their provider organization. As this relationship grows, so will the quality of the relationship between these providers and the individual patients they serve.

As this change begins to take place, patients will find it easier to say to physicians, "With all due respect, Doctor, when you poke me with that cold instrument without telling me what you are doing, I don't feel good about it." Growing up means increasing overall quality because bedside manner is not purely a matter of marketing or PR; it is an aspect of the process of healing, which is the purpose for the relationship in the first place. Actively seeking and remaining open to, and accepting of, such feedback isn't easy when the profession and its patients have together created an ethos that attributes godliness to human beings who have earned the legitimate title of medical expert.

Physician-executives have a unique contribution to make. They have been members of the fraternity. They can empathize with the pain of slung arrows. People such as Ray Fernandez understand the dynamics of patient-provider anxiety and dependence. They know it in their heart and soul. As they earn the legitimate expertise of educated professional managers, they will be in a position to help build the bridges of transition essential to their organization's growing up.

The bridges I see as necessary will take the form of building new interpersonal relationships. I believe that all communication is an attempt at social influence. A picture of these new, synergistic relationships can be developed using the template of the *push* and *pull* styles of communication introduced earlier.[28] Power and influence as dynamic processes, messages, take place or are carried out through communications.

The content of an expert's push behaviors would be primarily *descriptive* and *prescriptive:* "I suggest you take this medication twice daily for two weeks because you

---

[28] See p. 40.

have symptoms A, B, and C, and this drug is highly effective in these cases." "You need to extend office hours into the evening and weekends because our patient satisfaction surveys show this as a priority need." If experts with a priestly mien believe that it is their divine right to pontificate without explanation, prescriptions offered without clear, detailed, descriptive reasons or explanations will likely result.

An expert's *pull* behaviors would be narrowly confined to *attending* (listening) and *asking*. The *asking* would be very specific, for example, "Do you have any questions about my prescription?" "Have you completed your department's five-year plan yet?" Here again, if an expert's ego has gotten out of hand, impatience creeps in, and *attending* behaviors get cut short.

A team, adult-to-adult relationship does not eliminate the above, but rather expands it in terms of styles of behavior. The expert enthusiastically and openly *asks* for suggestions: "What do you think is causing the problem? How have you considered changing the situation?" Since the patient would have an equal role in the relationship, the physician would exhibit more *understanding* behaviors: (a) to the patient "So what you're telling me is, you tend to skip breakfast and lunch regularly," and (b) to a colleague: "Our disagreement seems to stem from my needing to have 24-hour coverage and your not wanting to take any night call." Of course, true teamwork is impossible without mutual respect and empathy.

Comparable changes would be seen on the *push* side. The patient (or employee) and the expert (physician or manager) would both be offering prescriptions, suggestions, to improve the situation. Explanations of descriptive facts and reasons would be detailed, in language the *receiver* could understand, and would be offered willingly, not grudgingly. An educated, knowledgeable patient or employee is a valuable asset.

Such rebalancing, realignment, and reattunement will be very difficult for people intent on sailing in the narrow channels of expert power. I emphasize that each party has the power to be 100% responsible for their part in the relationship. If patients change their behavior with their doctors, then the relationship with their doctors will be different. If the doctors are more informative with their patients, then their relationship with their patients will be different. When the Nalle Clinic began to change its relationship with its physician-staff, some left because they liked the old way better.

There is a price to these changes: vulnerability. Dr. Berman said it well:

> Acknowledging their expertise and your own deficiencies and asking for their help are critical and are not—as might be initially feared—at all inconsistent with the authoritative style recommended earlier. Confidence and strength are required to know and own one's limitations. Since people expect physicians to be egotists, a bit of honest humility goes a long way—especially when the truth of such an attitude is so apparent.[29]

---

[29] See p. 56.

Bluffing, a *push* behavior motivated by fear, gets interpreted as arrogance; and it increases others' resistance. Acknowledging our own deficiencies reduces our own and others' fears, clearing the path for change. As the old adage goes, the truth sets us free. Stage-III organizations, as we have noted, engage people's souls. That's powerful! Because they feel such a deep level of involvement in the business and little unmanageable fear, people have little difficulty "doing whatever needs to be done."[30]

Perhaps the greatest change in the behavioral communication patterns would be seen in the area of feedback: *appreciate* behavior and very specific *asks*. People sincerely motivated to improve the quality of any relationship must be continuously aware of their own behavior and consequences. Until an organization is at Stage III, where members see themselves as being in partnership, the person in the high-power position must take the lead in periodically *asking*, "How is my behavior affecting the quality of our relationship from your point of view?" "What am I doing, intentionally or not, that could lead you to conclude that I do not care for you?"

It will take time to overcome the anxiety and fear associated with an authority asking this question *and* a patient (in the broadest sense of the word), answering it with assertive authority.

Physicians will maintain their expert power over matters of technical quality. Patients have expertise over a different domain. Lacking medical competence, patients "must rely on the affective dimension [TLC] of the doctor-patient relationship in evaluating the physician's role performances."[31] But over time, it is this feedback process that is the lifeblood of change and growth in any relationship. Without feedback there is no growing up, no increasing teamwork.

The more the ambiguity, the greater the fear and anxiety we feel. The bridge we must have, especially during transitions, is the helping hand of staying in touch, feeling the pulse. The greater the ambiguity, the closer must be the contact, just as ships in a fog must sound their horns more frequently.

When the sailing got rough at the Nalle Clinic, trusted physician colleagues jumped ship. An observer commented, "All they're thinking about is what's going to be important to them, no matter who they step on or let down."[32]

TLC without all the available technology will only prolong patient suffering. On the other hand, technology without the power of TLC carries little hope for the healing profession to be able to first heal itself.[33]

Our only hope may lie in the hands and hearts of men and women like Dr. Ray

---

[30] See p. 22 for further discussion of attaining organizational excellence.

[31] Press, p. 54.

[32] See p. 91 for full quotation.

[33] For a discussion of technology and TLC, high tech/high touch, see John Naisbitt, *Megatrends: Ten New Directions Transforming Our Lives,* (New York: Warner Books, 1982).

Fernandez who have the courage to struggle to guide their institutions through the turbulent passages of growing up.

So the stage is set for the most familiar confrontation of modern life— between people who demand change and institutions who resist it. The institutions alter, but never fast enough, and those who seek change are bitterly disappointed.

In the resulting conflict we find our institutions in a savage crossfire between uncritical lovers and unloving critics. On the one side those who love their institutions tend to smother them in an embrace of death. On the other side there has arisen a breed of critics without love, skilled in demolition and untutored in the arts by which human institutions are nurtured and strengthened and made to flourish. Where human institutions are concerned, love without criticism brings stagnation and criticism without love brings destruction. The swifter the pace of change, the more lovingly men must care for and criticize their institutions to keep them intact through the turbulent passages.[34]

---

[34] John Gardner, *Recovery of Confidence,* (New York: W.W. Norton Co., Inc., 1970), pp. 29–30.

Part Four:

Closure and Prognosis

CHART ENTRY:
ENDINGS AND BEGINNINGS

by Irwin Rubin, Ph.D.

A transformation that began years ago—that had allowed Dr. Fernandez to accept an entire organization of providers as his primary-care patients— was entering its next stage. His struggle to accept the painful realization that he was about to become the first former physician-CEO of the Nalle Clinic reflects the human experience of death and dying at two levels: the first, the loss of title or position, seemed minor next to the second. The really painful deaths are those associated with losing the respect and friendship of longstanding colleagues. Following one's heart and doing what you deeply believe is best for the welfare of the whole will not always result in remaining popular. To better understand this aspect of leadership, we will need to draw lessons from the agony of defeat as well as from the thrill of victory. To broaden our conscious awareness and insight, we must venture into what Jung calls the shadow side of our own personalities.

I made a special effort to stay in touch with Dr. Fernandez during this period of turmoil and upheaval, a period he anticipated, although he did not anticipate its emotional intensity. He describes it in the closing paragraph of his personal chart entry of December 5, 1988:

> The highs are higher and the lows, lower in my current position than in medical practice. As patients literally put their lives in their physician's hands, so the life of the organization is in mine. The challenge of controlling a complex organization's culture, financial performance, quality control, and morale is exciting. As the organization progresses through change and growth, I take a parent's pride in its successes. Still, the fear and frustration of dealing with the unknown is something physician-managers have to live with every day. Like Columbus, we have to realize that most people actually hope we'll fall off the end of the world so that they can remain secure in their belief that the world is flat, and that physicians do not make good administrators.

In addition to wanting to support an old friend and colleague, I knew from my experience and training that some of the hostility toward him reflected normal transference dynamics of the leadership process. When your patient is a gangling adolescent, you expect and recognize the need for an intense period of counter-dependence. He'll sass you and think you're from the Stone Age, but you realize that it's all part of his process of accepting responsibilities and becoming an interdependent

RY

adult. As John Gardner recently put it in an interview, "For any leader, there is an absolutely unresolvable tension between the responsibilities to those he or she leads, and the responsibilities to the greater good." As a consequence, Gardner concludes, one of the unrecognized qualities leaders must develop is the capacity to absorb hostility, "to learn not to take it personally, to realize the criticism is aimed at the office, not at them."[35]

However, while the rational mind knows that the child must struggle to make its own way, the heart still experiences the pain of the separation. In a January 24, 1990, letter, Dr. Fernandez expressed his feelings: "Tough time to go through right now—feelings of loneliness, lack of appreciation, confusion, and failure. Must be like living through a divorce!" The emotional closeness, the bonding which takes place between physician and patient, was beginning to shift. In addition, colleagues who disagreed with his leadership were jumping ship, taking valued affiliations, business and personal, with them. The image of divorce aptly captures this process. Long after the formal decrees are signed, it's painful when divorced partners bump into one another.

In January 1990 the discontent at the Nalle Clinic received a public airing. Dr. Fernandez wrote, "Have included a few clippings FYI [for your information]. [Quotes from *Business Journal* and *Observer* appear in commentary in Part Three.] Media isn't *helping* me to keep morale and trust up! Got to admit that this is the low point of an otherwise fine career in management. Interesting to observe how some 'old friends' ignore the painful situation, others simply acknowledge it, and others express concern and support."

To come to terms with the feeling that he was losing his patient and valued colleagues—the pain of impending divorce, to which he previously referred—I suggested to Dr. Fernandez that he talk about these feelings with his wife and that he tape-record these conversations. The chart entries I have selected for this fourth part of our clinical analysis will be brief excerpts from private encounters between Dr. and Mrs. Fernandez. As readers, we are privileged to glimpse these conversations, for they can help us see aspects of the leadership process that we might overlook.

I must approach my interpretive commentary, which I will interweave with the chart entries rather than following our previous format, even more cautiously than in Part Two. As you have become aware, my psychological bias is Jungian. In this context, for any healing to be complete, masculine and feminine perceptions must be in harmony. In the Jungian sense, these terms reflect archetypal qualities in every person—not gender-specific qualities. That means, each of us is a composite of intellect and feeling, intuition and rational thought, toughness and softness, masculine and feminine. Conscious awareness of new beginnings and endings often resonate

---

[35] Joe Flower, "The Role of the Leader," *Healthcare Forum Journal,*" May/June 1990, p. 33.

as the stirring of feelings arising from the feminine. We are fortunate to be able to include in our final chart entries the perspectives from Mrs. Gail Fernandez. She's a catalyst, a behind-the-scenes confidante, and a supporter of his transformation from physician to physician-manager to physician-CEO.

Early in the first of these conversations, Mrs. Fernandez is recounting a phone conversation she had with the wife of a physician who had just announced his resignation from the Clinic. While having "no hard feelings against" the husband's needing to "go his own way," Mrs. Fernandez also "felt a real sense of lack of loyalty." In spite of the thought that "I'm sure they're the same people," she reported that the quality of their relationship "seems to have changed. As a result, I had a strained feeling." Mrs. Fernandez, too, has lost an old friendship.

The masculine part of ourselves that allows us to feel married to a career might find it difficult to maintain psychic boundaries between achievement and affiliation, between business and friendship. (In our society, this part is usually stronger in men.) The feminine side (which is usually stronger in women), typically puts relationships before personal achievement. Mrs. Fernandez reports that "these problems have not been as difficult for me [as they were for Dr. Fernandez]. I've been able, for the most part, to separate Clinic from personal. Most of my friends have been able to see me apart from the Clinic problems of their spouses. Two or three friendships have, unfortunately, been totally ended—on their part, not mine."

When we betray the precarious psychic balance between our short-term self-interest and our joint commitment to a long-term relationship, our feminine side screams out. If we violate our own values on the path to success, our success feels meaningless. We sit at the top, empty. The process of leadership carries both the joys of life and the pains of death.

In exploring more deeply her own unease regarding physicians who deserted during the time of stress, Mrs. Fernandez comments to her husband,

> I just feel like they were looking out for their own benefit, which I guess I can't fault them with. But they jumped ship, not thinking about how the rest of us felt that were still a part of the Nalle Clinic, but just concerned to look out for themselves. And to me, in a nutshell, that's what's happening: these guys aren't looking at a group practice, or a clinic that they need to be loyal to as players of a team. All they're thinking about is what's going to be important to them—no matter who they step on or let down.
>
> Well, I'm sure they blame you. I'm sure they've said many harsh words about you in their homes or with whoever they can talk to about the Clinic. That's hard for me to understand, because you're a tool of the Clinic. You're only an agent of the Clinic who's supposed to carry out its mission. So I can't understand why it's your fault.

In labeling the fears lurking in the shadow of her husband's psyche—the possibility, horrifying to any physician, that he might have been guilty of malpractice in the care of his patient—and in bringing out into the open words others spoke in the shadows behind his back, Mrs. Fernandez enables Dr. Fernandez to begin the painful acceptance of his new role, with its diminished responsibilities and authority. Just as his colleagues felt he had betrayed them when he moved from physician to physician-manager to physician-CEO, he now feels his patient is betraying *him* as it moves away from him.

The first stages in dealing with death and dying—denial and anger—become immediately accessible to the psyche when the feminine can speak so the masculine can hear. Dr. Fernandez writes,

> They pushed me. . . . They gave me the helm of this ship, albeit not a very seaworthy craft. They forget the fact that what they're asking for is unreasonable, or perhaps even impossible to accomplish *[just as, in the heat of the moment, Dr. Fernandez forgets the fact that he took the helm without a clear job description or a set of performance indicators]*. They don't realize that the captain needs money, staff, and the support of a crew to sail.

Notwithstanding that the criticism is not personal but a part of the turf (leaving aside the question of whether it is justifiable), it hurts. Denial and anger are natural human responses. Learning to deal with hostility does not mean becoming impervious to the pain, for then leaders risk losing the acute sensitivity necessary to feel the pulse of their constituency. The leader must manage the pain and find safe outlets for discharging it.

Sensitive to Dr. Fernandez's anger and hurt, and with the feminine's sense of our inherent interdependence, Mrs. Fernandez reminds him of the impossibility of sailing a ship when "everybody's jumping overboard." "It can't be done overnight," she adds, especially "when they don't give you all the essential tools." The feminine knows well that children grow up only in their own time, requiring constant attention, feeding, and nurturing.

Feeling "like a failure, like I'm not doing a good job" begins to come into balance with Dr. Fernandez's ability to see and accept what he is experiencing. He gets conscious and unconscious contradictory messages: on the one hand, that he "is important, that the organization recognizes and knows it needs its leader"; on the other hand, this same organization says, "We don't want you; it's time for a new administration."

As Dr. Fernandez becomes painfully aware, leadership during periods of cultural transition is full of mixed signals saying, "You're damned if you do and damned if you don't." Realizing that it's not personal enables him to resist the temptation to "bail out . . . go on and do something else that might feel personally better." Instead, he realizes that quality patient care means eliminating himself as physician-CEO. In other words, he refers his patient, the Nalle Clinic, to another specialist.

This phase of leadership in organizational cultural change is physically and emotionally demanding. There are tough settlements to make. The impending joint venture with PhyCor—the transition to a Stage-II business organization—requires Dr. Fernandez to negotiate termination agreements with valued colleagues and old friends who did not choose to stay with PhyCor. We can understand that physicians are reluctant to perform complicated surgery on family and close friends. Similarly, when your patient is an entire organization in the midst of cultural change, in the "turning over of the reins of management and decision-making to new people," you will inevitably and reluctantly have to tell some dear, old friends that their membership is terminal. Whispered rumors, totally unfounded, that those in leadership positions are accepting under-the-table sweeteners do not make the dirty work of leadership any easier. The feminine jumps to the fore at this point, and Mrs. Fernandez labels that dynamic for what it is, a natural projection from shadows of anxious psyches: "That's their motivation, but that is not your motivation." Thus, although he finds this pettiness frustrating, Dr. Fernandez is able to acknowledge, "I guess there's no surprise."

As we bring this clinical case to a close, I must reemphasize a point I made in the commentary to Part Two: "[I]t is individuals who act as leaders. Whether or not these initiatives are mutually beneficial, and at what costs to whom, depend on the quality of the exchange. The quality of the partnership, the relationship between a patient and a provider, determines the outcome of healing."

Just as pieces of Dr. Fernandez's self-image had to change in order for him to transform his commitment to patient care to an entire organization, so, too, the organization—his patient—had to experience the loss of an old identity to take on a new one. Both parties to the leadership relationship have to experience their versions of the natural cycles of beginnings and endings. Although we read Dr. Benedum's view in the commentaries in Part Three, we do not know how the entire patient-organization would describe its experiences of leadership and organizational cultural change as it struggled to grow up.

We do know that 48 hours after the PhyCor negotiations closed, a previously scheduled Nalle Clinic annual party took place. The timing of this symbolic act of breaking bread, which Dr. Fernandez attributes to "just an absolute stroke of providence," Jung would have seen as pure synchronicity.

Instead of the depression of the past few months, Dr. Fernandez reports an "amazing turn when people knew where we were going. . . . There was no longer any question about who was in and who was out." A renewed sense of pride seemed to surge through the patient, a feeling as if "we had really succeeded almost beyond our wildest dreams." Handshaking and back patting replaced finger pointing and back stabbing. People were "starting to smile again." Even the press acknowledged the positive momentum that had begun. Within two months, a prestigious family-practice group of eleven physicians in four satellites joined the Clinic.

Even the solitary individual who, in the face of growing dissension and desertion, had led the patient where the patient wanted to go[36] reported "actually getting . . . some congratulations." One of his colleagues captured the essence of leadership (the dirty work) in organizational cultural change, when he congratulated Dr. Fernandez on being able "to turn chicken shit into chicken salad."

Epilogue

Writing on the perils of detachment in the health-care industry, Emily Friedman describes the "basic conflict of the care giver: 'How can I be compassionate without becoming so involved that I cannot bear the suffering?'" She warns us, "When patients cease to be people, everything is lost."[37] Living on the horns of this dilemma—when your patient is an entire organization—is one of the leadership challenges. In this unedited last paragraph of the tape dictated several days after the annual party, Dr. Fernandez reminds us all of the essential lesson of humility at the core of leadership and organizational cultural change.

> I guess it must be like the general in times of war having to order some of his troops to storm the hill, absolutely knowing full well in advance that a lot of them are going to get shot and killed. When knowing that that's what's necessary to win the war—you've got to lose some of your people in battle. I guess still the general doesn't sleep very well at night, knowing that his command is what causes a lot of very, very personal suffering. Even though maybe it's his army that ultimately prevails and wins the war.

---

[36] 99.5% of the Clinic's physicians voted to sell their shares to PhyCor.
[37] "The Perils of Detachment," *Healthcare Forum Journal*," March/April 1990, p. 10.

COMMENTARY:
"WHAT'S IT ALL ABOUT, ALFIE?"

by Dr. Raymond Fernandez
August 1990

W hat does all this change and the effect that it had on me and the organization really mean? What are the lessons here? Those close to me are asking how things are going now, six months into a very new structure at the Clinic. To a casual observer, my role has changed significantly. But candidly, in a crucial way it hasn't changed at all. I have always been asked to be an interpreter and a commentator. A crucial duty I have performed all along is to help those around me who were actually performing the work of the organization to understand what the organization is doing and how their role is meaningful. Right now that interpreter's function is more crucial than ever.

Not only my role, but everyone's role in the organization has changed. I'm but an indicator of how things are. It's a truism that during times of transition and evolution, those in the middle of change may have a hard time seeing that things are changing around them. The many false starts and brief stops of our organization, when viewed over a continuum of time, have been very hard emotionally on the individuals primarily involved in those changes. But physicians always see their patients episodically. A patient's only doctor visit for a while might be for an annual physical examination. If so, the physician can easily lose sight that the patient has a life between doctor visits and, indeed, that that individual's life is outside of the doctor's office. The sick patient who is hospitalized again is visited only briefly and episodically by the physician. It is only over the continuum of years that the patient's true health status can be assessed. The physician easily gets emotionally involved and empathic with the patient during times of diagnosed crises. But the best role for the physician and patient can only be worked out when the physician sees the patient's life moving forward—occasionally with assistance from the physician, sometimes in spite of the physician, but most importantly, progressing best when the patient takes on responsibility for his or her own health. Both doctor and patient must resist the temptation that the patient become dependent on the physician.

It was in September of 1989 that maximum stresses were occurring within the organization. I can't help but recall the ironic analogy that struck Charlotte, North Carolina at that same time in the form of Hurricane Hugo. This was one of the most devastating storms to hit the United States in history. Who could have expected so much destruction, especially 200 miles inland? The city of Charlotte was left without electricity for weeks, with a snarled transportation system, inability of businesses to open their doors, and untold property damage. One of Charlotte's proudest assets is its stately trees, and fully 25% of them were lost. The unexpected tempest resulted in loss of all the weaker trees. Those with a deep, strong root system endured and now prosper. But the temporary change in the topography was soon cleared, and the scars left on a lovely city were removed by the proud citizens who remained and rolled up their sleeves.

The Clinic used its internal tempest as a time to restructure, reassess, and refocus. An outside agency (PhyCor) served as the necessary emergency vehicle that came to the assistance of a neighbor. PhyCor represented an outside resource that could be called upon to help make certain needed changes and to shore up certain bent, but not broken, trees. The Clinic had previously been thinking of a new structure to improve decision making and to promote leadership. It had brought non-physicians onto its Board of Directors. It was considering giving ownership over to a tax-free foundation. It had recognized its adolescent growing pains. It only required—and, indeed, provided itself—an emergency to force actions that might otherwise have been postponed.

Now six months into a new structure, it is obvious that certain goals that eluded us in the past could now be accomplished almost with ease. We have changed our compensation formula. We have altered pension benefits to be more realistic. A reserve fund is established, and a profit margin is being obtained. Marketing is being planned in earnest.

Physicians now feel a much greater sense of security than they have had in a good while. They are able to get back to the basics. Their concentration is now on practicing medicine, and they have more confidence that the administrative aspects and the control of overhead will be taken care of. They don't find it necessary to have the direct personal involvement in this, as they did before. Thus, the physicians have given up some of their control. But the tradeoff has more than made up for any loss: Physicians now feel comfortable going about their primary task of providing medical services to patients.

My personal sense through this is that I, too, have given up a large element of control of the Clinic. It is a pleasure watching us being more successful than ever before. It's as though now I'm watching someone else being successful at something I started. The patient that was last seen in intensive care and had to be referred out to a specialist is now back in full health. There is a sense of pride that now we are meeting certain goals that had to be met. That accomplishment is much more important than bickering about which administration is accomplishing it.

Editor's Note: In a tape he dictated just prior to the manuscript's going to press, Dr. Fernandez provided an additional and critical insight as to an important and normal aspect of what this process of organizational growing up is all about. For six weeks he had pushed for an annual performance evaluation (critical, as we noted earlier, to the growing-up process), in his continuing role as full-time Medical Director.

"The two officers [of the Board] assigned the task of doing this job," he reports, "gave me an excellent evaluation." In their proposal to the Board, however, they were going to recommend "that the amount of time devoted by the Medical Director to administrative duties should decrease from 'a full-time job' to 65 percent." In addition to finding that personally unacceptable, Dr. Fernandez knew that such regression, while not unusual, was potentially dangerous: "It seemed to me like a patient who was over an acute illness and no longer in pain, jumping to the conclusion that they didn't need as much medical care."

In no uncertain terms, Dr. Fernandez informed his patient of the risks involved. "I pointed out that it is premature to declare victory," that in spite of the essential support that PhyCor offered, "it would be a step backward to diminish the time, knowledge, energy, and commitment of the Clinic to promoting its own internal systems [to growing up]." The Medical Director, Dr. Fernandez stressed, "functions as a personification of the Board of Directors itself and represents the spirit of the leadership team." To diminish the role—as a principle, independent of personalities—he warns the patient, "would be to diminish the role of the Board of Directors and the entire leadership of the Clinic." Such loving toughness, though difficult to manifest, is absolutely essential. Fortunately, it "got their attention," for after a "vigorous discussion, the Board unanimously reaffirmed that they still want a full-time Medical Director with appropriate compensation."

This little vignette confirms what we knew all along about the process of growing up. Perfection (perfect health) is an abstraction that lives only in mythology. Physical, emotional, intellectual, and spiritual progress is all we humans can claim. As Dr. Fernandez concluded, "The battle is never really over."

COMMENTARY: HUMAN PARALLELS TO ORGANIZATIONAL DEVELOPMENT

by Irwin Rubin, Ph.D.

*I*n the Nalle Clinic we can find many human parallels to normal organizational development as I have described it in the commentary "Organizations Have to Grow Up." I don't know of any widely accepted, empirically verified model of the growth stages that people in organizations go through. The mission of the health-care industry depends on a human process. Skilled professionals use all human and technological means available to heal patients. Humanization of this industry is not (as might be true in the automobile industry, for example), simply a matter of altruism ("It's good to be good to people"), or business profitability. When the bottom line is healing, treating people with TLC (tender love and care), is essential. Humanness in health care is the heart and soul of the business. Humanness is the values and behaviors that inspire commitment to quality care, to healing. A humanistic model of organizational development in health care could contribute to the development of a more humanistic industry and higher-quality patient care.

There is an intimate relationship between the organizations that comprise an industry and the industry as a whole. By examining the development of the Nalle Clinic, we can see what is going on in other organizations and in the health-care industry. (Similarly, by looking at these, we can learn about other industries.) Both the Clinic and the health-care industry mature through a series of stages. Both have a mission or direction. Both must reexamine their fundamental purpose. Until this mission work is completed, neither will be able to develop new solutions to problems of structure and procedure.

In labeling a Stage-I health-care organization as having a "childlike orientation," I did not mean to suggest that individual members are themselves childlike. They are seriously dedicated to the care of patients. The term describes the quality of the relationships, particularly among the physicians and between them and their parent organization. I do not use it judgmentally; I use it to describe a normal developmental process. Learning to walk is a prerequisite to gaining the strength, balance, and sense of purpose, to run.

Within Maslow's developmental hierarchy of human motivation, the parent organization provides the fraternity membership a roof overhead, food on the table, and protection against external threat, particularly these days from the legal fraternity. Consistent with the spirit of a childlike orientation, the members of the fraternity expect to receive these benefits at the lowest possible cost. They resist spending for the long-term improvement of the frat house because to do so would mean fewer dollars to gratify their personal needs now.

Once there was a physician who fancied himself as a medical George Patton, complete with "a pearl-handled stethoscope." He imagined he could lead his fraternal colleagues onto innovative beachheads in medicine. Any readers with teenagers will recognize their own family dynamic in his description of the difference between reality and fantasy:

> He said the difference between the Patton image and the reality of his medical leadership could be exemplified by a typical meeting in which (1) three of the people critical to the meeting and whom he counted on to provide support would arrive late; (2) two other key physicians would argue vigorously against the concept that he was proposing; (3) several other physicians indicated that they would not be at all interested in participating in the program; and (4) one physician would indicate that unless he was authorized to expend more money on specialized equipment for traditional programs, he would not participate in any new efforts by the organization (but would be willing to head a committee to organize the purchase of the equipment).[38]

We never resolve our developmental issues once and for all. They keep coming back. Discussing the psychosocial hurdles we must clear during our lives, Erikson carefully points out that new experiences will unsettle once-satisfactory levels of developmental achievement.[39] For example, while learning a new skill, adults naturally feel like babes in the woods. In Erikson's terms, we will reexperience the autonomy challenge, which we first confronted in our childhood. Similarly, seriously ill patients will feel the fear and dependency that go along with the basic trust hurdle we all faced in infancy.

This notion of natural regression helps us understand the developmental challenges that health care faces as an industry. In Erikson's framework, organized medicine is in its infancy or early childhood. Whereas individual professionals have passed at least once through many of Erikson's stages, the industry as a whole has not yet done so.

George Bernard Shaw noted, "The tragedy of illness at present is that it delivers you helplessly into the hands of a profession which you deeply mistrust." This comment speaks directly to Erikson's first developmental challenge of infancy, the trust

---

[38] André L. Delbecq and Sandra L. Gill, "Justice as a Prelude to Teamwork in Medical Centers," *HCM Review*, Winter, 1985, p. 46.

[39] Erik Erikson, *Childhood and Society*, Second Edition, (New York: W.W. Norton & Company, Inc., 1964).

issue. The idea that the "air of the operating room, where once the doctor was sovereign, is now so dense with the second guesses of insurers, regulators, lawyers, consultants, and risk managers that the physician has little room to breathe, much less heal," speaks directly to Erikson's second developmental challenge of autonomy. The *Time* magazine article that reported these comments was quick to point out that "the soreness may also reflect the stresses and strains of a profession in transition."[40]

Individuals cannot detour around developmental hurdles. If we try to stay put, we risk stagnating. The same is true for health-care organizations and the industry they are a part of. Group-practice organizations, in particular, will have to work through some aspects of the fraternity model. This training will develop the strength and perspective necessary to become a Stage-II business organization.

While each organization must chart its own course through Stage II, the waters have been navigated before. And many have lived to tell and write the tale. The basic business organization is a highly researched, well-documented organism. Scientists have done much ground-breaking research on adult roles, needs, and performance. Seasoned travelers offer regular trainings through health-care associations.

I don't doubt that the health-care industry will rise to the challenges of adolescence and young adulthood and get down to business. But the real challenge is yet to come. An industry whose fundamental mission requires individual members to "give up a piece of their *souls*—to invest their *selves* in the business"—has no choice but to become replete with Stage-III organizations. It's not enough for the health-care industry to have well-run businesses. No, not in a healing profession. As I said earlier, the search for excellence is the foundation of the entire profession of medicine. Physicians are always working to improve patient care with a more effective laser, antibiotic, or diet. Continuous improvement is equally critical when the patient is an entire organization of providers.

Because the industry is young, few Stage-III organizations are available for study, although many organizations are preparing themselves for the push to the next plateau. Deming-and-Juran-type projects, which focus on technical quality assurance and cost savings, can contribute to creating strong Stage-II health-care organizations. In my experience, their left-brain focus does not speak to the non-linear, quantum leap in consciousness necessary to propel us into the search for excellence. Both the quality and the discussion of the information that individuals contribute in their quality circles rest upon the highest levels of trust. While Deming's steps refer to the need to reduce fear, in my own experience, few organizations treat this issue with the attention it deserves.

Health-care institutions exist to fulfill two functions: curative and healing. Curing

[40] Nancy Gibbs, "Sick and Tired," *Time*, July 31, 1989, pp. 48–9.

requires technical effectiveness (trained providers performing skillfully) and managerial efficiency (the organization must survive financially to fulfill any function). Healing, by contrast, requires love and nurturance, heart and soul (versus mind and matter). Total quality care is a function of three factors: effectiveness, efficiency, and TLC.

Continuous improvement through experiential learning requires overcoming the debilitating effects of fear and anxiety. Just as the fear of dying can sap a patient's strength and will to live, the fear of negative treatment from within the organization can sap a provider's strength and capacity to care. For example, a board of trustees that removes a CEO in an inhumane manner, and thus traumatizes the provider organization, can infect the healing culture of its organization. And angry physicians who verbally abuse nursing staff (or medical students, as recent research[41] has suggested), may be guilty of behavioral malpractice as poisonous, and as avoidable, as staph infections in the operating room.

Love and nurturance, the seeds from which healing experiences grow, are human commodities that health-care institutions must produce before they can share. Like other treasured natural resources, TLC is not a commodity that we can abuse without replenishing. We can't buy it and stock it on the shelf. It must be given freely and, like a child's spontaneity, it will only be sustained by an environment free of unwarranted fear and anxiety, by a healing culture.[42] As St. Marguerite Hospital in Japan has learned, treating patients, be they individuals or organizations, with TLC is the way to reduce fear.

The search for excellence requires continuous learning from experience. Still, each succeeding cycle will confront new and unfamiliar territory. Unless we regularly experience feeling like "babes in the woods," we cannot be certain we are sailing, as Columbus did, on heretofore uncharted waters. If we are, we need new skills. Our lunar astronauts faced this Columbus-like challenge. No human experience existed that would help them prepare for a forced landing on the dark side of the moon, cut off from earth communication. Training for that possibility involved learning how to use consensual decision-making (as opposed to traditionally relying on their commander) to become map makers. Map-reading skills would have been useless in an emergency.

This line of thinking aligns the challenges of human development and organizational development. First, the very fear and anxiety that patients experience when they are seriously ill is no different from the fear and anxiety that health-care organizations experience as they set sail in search of excellence. Second, just as self-actu-

---

[41] Silver and Glicken, pp. 527–537.

[42] Excerpted from an unpublished article by Irwin Rubin, "Managing Fear and Its Effects on the Quality of Care," copyright 1990 by Temenos®, Inc., U.S.A.

alization is an ideal in human development, excellence is an ideal in organizational development.

In an article about the respected medical futurist Leland Kaiser, Wesley Curry writes,

> A paradox for the next century will be that, as we move to high technology, we will also move to high touch. . . . One of the important distinctions to make in the years ahead in terms of medical care is the difference between curing and healing. . . . Curing is a problem for medical science. Healing is a problem of human love and nurturance. . . .
>
> Dr. Kaiser expects healing to play a greater role in the system in the future. "I think the hospital of the future will say that it heals everyone who comes through its doors. Those it can cure, it cures." Dr. Kaiser calls this new hospital an "experiential organization." He says that it provides a "transforming experience" for the patient.[43]

According to our fundamental premise, the health-care organization of the future will provide a "transforming experience" for patients only to the extent that it provides a transforming experience for its own members. To enhance the quality of the healing experience the industry offers patients, it will first have to heal itself. I don't mean to imply a current state of illness; rather, I am speaking of yet another attempt to grow up.

Malpractice mania is rampant. As a result, many practicing physicians feel despair, wishing they had never gone into medicine in the first place. With college students choosing other professions, medical-school enrollments have dropped. While these industry trends are painful, they can signal a basic, and ultimately strengthening, developmental transition.

What will it take to grow up? First, Erikson's challenge to the medical industry involves a willingness to reach out and seek enrichment from its patients. He says that humans are a teaching and a learning animal.[44] Part of the problem of mistrust between physicians and patients is that there hasn't been enough give and take. So far, it's been mostly give from the physicians and mostly take from the patients. Just as parents learn from and teach their children, providers and patients are interdependent, too. While we cannot, and should not, expect lay patients to be able to judge the quality of the technical care they receive, the patients should be the final authority on the quality of the human care they receive.

Second, there must be a healing attitude—by this I mean human love and nurturance—in the whole organization: among administrators, physicians, and staff. (In

---

43. Wesley Curry, "Looking Ahead," *Physician Executive*, 16, no. 1, (January–February 1990), p. 4.
44. Erikson, p. 216.

the past, the healing attitude has usually been from physicians toward their patients.) The adversarial attitude between administrators has made it difficult for physicians to treat their patients with love and nurturance. A squabble in the meeting room does not make for kindness in the treatment room. Providers who, in the short run, manage to put squabbles out of their minds and to be the ideal healers to their patients, face early burnout. TLC is a human commodity that a health-care organization must generate before it can export it to patients. As Emily Friedman warned, "When patients cease to be people, everything is lost."[45] We must remember the plaque outside St. Marguerite Hospital that promises

 To heal sometimes
To support often
To comfort always

George Bernard Shaw's comment, referred to earlier, that "The tragedy of illness at present is that it delivers you helplessly into the hands of professionals you deeply mistrust" challenges the health-care industry to regain a rapidly eroding sense of integrity. Integrity means keeping its mission in mind—that is, being primarily concerned with the patient's well being. I remember our family doctor, who brought me into the world and all my sisters, too. He was *our* doctor. My parents wouldn't have dreamed of suing him, because they knew how much he cared for us. Nowadays, some patients think their doctors care more for money. Patients wonder why they're being sent for another test. Perhaps his colleagues need the business? Perhaps the doctor is practicing defensive medicine, fearing a lawsuit? In either case, the motive for the test is not believed to be love for the patient. To rise to a Stage-III organization, to self-actualize, means, in Erikson's terms, to win another round in the constant human battle of despair vs. ego integrity. An industry that possesses integrity "is ready to defend the dignity of its own mission against all physical and economic threats."[46]

What will happen to organizations that do not choose to change? Staying in Stage I means remaining a fraternity, at least for a while. Obsolescence is the most likely long-term consequence. Stagnation in Stage II is not likely to be fatal to the organization. Neither will it result in the fullest healing of its patients.

By developing a humanistic organizational paradigm that acknowledges the essential oneness of human development with organizational development, the health-care industry has the opportunity to contribute to the health of the nation.

---

[45] Friedman, p. 10.

[46] Erikson, p. 268.

BIBLIOGRAPHY

Berwick, Donald. "Measuring Health Care Quality." *Pediatrics in Review,* 10 (1), (July 1988), 16.

Curry, Wesley. "Looking Ahead." *Physician Executive,* 16(1), (January–February 1990), 4.

Delbecq, André L., and Sandra L. Gill. "Justice as a Prelude to Teamwork in Medical Centers." *HCM Review,* Winter, 1985, 45–51.

Erikson, Erik. *Childhood and Society,* Second Edition. New York: W.W. Norton & Company, Inc., 1964.

Fernandez, Charles Raymond. "Personal Managerial Evolution in a Multispecialty Clinic." *Roads to Medical Management,* ed. Wesley Curry. Tampa: AAMD, 1988, 74–77.

Flower, Joe. "The Role of the Leader." *Healthcare Forum Journal,* (May/June 1990), 30–34.

French, John R. P., Jr., and Bertram Raven. "The Bases of Social Power," in *Group Dynamics: Research and Theory,* Third Edition, ed. Dorwin Cartwright and Alvin Zander. New York: Harper & Row, 1968, 263–268. Originally published in *Studies in Social Power.* D. Cartwright, ed. Ann Arbor, Mich.: Institute for Social Research, 1959.

Friedman, Emily. "The Perils of Detachment." *Healthcare Forum Journal,"* March/April 1990, 9–10.

Gardner, John. *Recovery of Confidence.* New York: W.W. Norton & Company, Inc., 1970, 29–30.

Gibbs, Nancy. "Sick and Tired." *Time,* July 31, 1989, 48–53.

Naisbitt, John. *Megatrends: Ten New Directions Transforming Our Lives.* New York: Warner Books, 1982.

Peters, Thomas J., and Robert H. Waterman, Jr. *In Search of Excellence.* New York: Harper & Row, 1982, 318–325.

Press, Irwin. "The Predisposition to File Claims: The Patient's Perspective." *Law, Medicine & Health Care,* (April 1984), 53–62.

Rubin, Irwin. "Organizations Have to Grow Up." *Physician Executive,* 13(2) (March–April 1987), 2–6.

Rubin, Irwin. "Managing Fear and Its Effects on the Quality of Care." Temenos®, Inc., U.S.A., 1990.

Rubin, Irwin, and Robert Inguagiato. "Behavioral Quality Assurance: A Transforming Experience." *Physician Executive,* 16(5), (Sept.–Oct. 1990), 30–33.

Schutte, James E. "An Impaired Doctor Cost his Colleagues $5 Million." *Medical Economics,* (June 4, 1990), 45–50.

Silver, Henry K., M.D., and Anita Duhl Glicken, M.S.W. "Medical Student Abuse: Incidence, Severity, and Significance." *JAMA,* 263(4), (January 26, 1990), 527–537.

To Order Additional Copies Of:

MY PULSE Is Not What It Used to Be:
The Leadership Challenges in Health Care

Write to:
The Temenos® Foundation
P.O. Box 37130
Honolulu, Hawaii 96837